INTERNATIONAL ASPECTS OF THE PROVISION
OF MEDICAL CARE

International Aspects

I I

of the

Provision of Medical Care

Edited by

P. W. KENT

Director, Glycoprotein Research Unit &
Master, Van Mildert College, Durham

ORIEL PRESS

STOCKSFIELD

LONDON — HENLEY ON THAMES — BOSTON

© 1976 Board of Management of the Foster & Wills Scholarships,
Oxford University, England

First published in 1976
by Oriel Press Ltd (Routledge & Kegan Paul Ltd)
Stocksfield, Northumberland, England NE43 7NA

Set in Linotype Juliana and
Printed in Great Britain by
Northumberland Press Limited, Gateshead

ISBN 0 85362 160 8

CONTENTS

CONTENTS

PREFACE

The chapters which constitute this volume arise out of contributions made at an international symposium held at Christ Church, Oxford in September 1974 under the general chairmanship of Sir George Pickering. The symposium was the third of its kind to be held under the auspices of the Board of Management of the Foster & Wills Scholarships at Oxford University and of the German Academic Exchange Service.

These Symposia, which occur annually, have subjects drawn alternately from the natural sciences and from the humanities, and it is a distinctive feature that their deliberations should be of an inter-disciplinary nature.

Both the symposium and this volume have been made possible by the most generous financial support of the Kulturabteilung of the German Foreign Office, the Stifterverband für die Deutsche Wissenschaft and the Deutscher Akademischer Austauschdienst. Particular thanks are due to Herr Risler, Herr Mruck, Mrs Farendon, the Steward of Christ Church, Mr E. M. James, and Dr J. M. Potter, for their contributions. Thanks are also due to A. M. Kent for preparing the index.

P. W. Kent
(general editor)
Van Mildert College
Durham

Chapter 1

A BACKGROUND OF HEALTH CARE PLANNING

T. McKEOWN
Medical School, University of Birmingham, England

IN BRITAIN, the public medical services evolved in the hundred years which preceded the introduction of the National Health Service. As in other countries, they were focussed initially on the problems of communicable disease, attacked by environmental measures and the provision of clinical services, including hospitals, for infectious patients. At the beginning of this century responsibility was extended into the field of personal health by the introduction of school and, later, maternal and child welfare services. In 1911 the first substantial commitment was made for therapeutic services by the National Health Insurance Act. Finally, in 1948, under the National Health Service (N.H.S.) public responsibility was accepted for all health services, financed mainly from taxation.

Critics of the NHS sometimes claimed that it changed radically the traditional pattern of medical services. It would be more accurate to say that it adopted with only minor modifications the framework of services which had evolved in the previous century. Important changes were the inevitable reduction of the amount of private practice and the transfer of responsibility for hospitals from local authorities. But general practice continued as before; hospital and consultant services were administered on the regional basis which developed during the second world war; and the traditional public health services were left with local government.

It would probably be agreed that the most tangible achievement of the service was to make medical care available to everyone and to remove the burden of direct payment from the large number of people who could ill afford it. In addition to this positive achievement it should be said that in the event many of the fears expressed about the public service proved to be groundless. It did not victimize doctors or public; it did not stifle initiative; it did not disturb the relationship between doctor and patient. The limitations were of a subtler kind, rooted in the tradition of health services.

From an administrative viewpoint, perhaps the most important limitation was that while the NHS was administered centrally by a single government department, local and regional responsibility was divided between three bodies. Hence there was no single authority with the duty and power to plan comprehensively, making the best use of resources according to a well judged scheme of priorities; moreover the framework of services divided hospital from domiciliary care and preventive from therapeutic medicine. Inevitably there were deficiencies, particularly in the domiciliary and community services, and in the case of the elderly, the disabled, the mentally ill and the mentally handicapped. There were also duplications, for example in obstetric and child health services which were divided between local authorities, general practitioners and hospitals.

In 1974 the NHS was revised in the light of the experience of quarter of a century. The main aim of the revision was the local and regional unification of responsibility for personal medical services. For reasons which need not be discussed here it was decided not to place the unified services under local government, and they have been assigned to new regional, area and district health authorities.

It should be recognized that the 1974 revision of the NHS was essentially administrative. It created a new framework within which the problems confronting health services can be tackled more effectively, but it did not resolve these problems. That is to say that unification of local and regional services should be seen as a necessary, rather than as a sufficient condition for future improvements; the major questions which confront health services everywhere have still to be answered. The remainder of this paper will be concerned with the background against which these questions might be considered and with a brief discussion of some of the more important issues.

THE BACKGROUND

Influences on health

Although the Hippocratic tradition gave due emphasis to other influences (for example, in *Airs, Waters and Places*), since the seventeenth century medical thought has been dominated by the belief that health depends primarily on an engineering approach, based on an understanding of the structure and function of the body and of the disease processes which affect it. This concept derives philosophically from Descartes, and appeared to find support in the work of Kepler and Harvey. It was thought to receive further confirmation in the success of the physical sciences, for it has been assumed that the approach which was so successful in modifying the physical environment could also be applied to living things, including man.

The effects of this conclusion in medicine are evident. Medical education begins with the study of the structure and functions of the body, continues with examination of disease processes and ends with clinical instruction on selected sick patients; medical service is dominated by the image of the acute hospital where the technological resources are concentrated; and medical science reflects the mechanistic concept, for example in the attention given to the chemical basis of inheritance and the immunological response to transplanted organs. These researches are strictly in accord with the Cartesian model, the first being thought to lead ultimately to control of gene structure and the second to replacement of diseased organs by normal ones. Hence the question is not whether the engineering approach is predominant in medicine, which would hardly be disputed, but whether it is seriously deficient as a conceptualization of the problems of human health. To answer this question it is necessary to examine the reasons for past improvements in health.

The modern transformation in man's health began in the eighteenth century. The evidence for this conclusion is the rapid growth of population, whose beginning cannot be dated exactly, but in Britain was probably in the first half of the century and in most western countries somewhat later. To account for the improvement in health it is therefore necessary to explain the modern rise of population.

Data for Sweden and England and Wales leave no doubt about two points: the growth of population resulted from a reduction of mortality; and the decline of mortality was due predominantly to a decrease in deaths from infectious diseases. There is no evidence of a reduction of non-infectious deaths before the present century, and they account for only about a tenth of the total decline of the death rate since the eighteenth century.

In interpreting the decline of the infections it seems right to dismiss at once the possibility that it was largely fortuitous, that it resulted from a change in the relationship between infectious organisms and man which was essentially independent of medical or other influences. Such changes undoubtedly occurred in relation to some organisms, for example the streptococcus whose variable virulence is attested by the well documented fluctuations of mortality from scarlet fever. But it is hardly credible that an explanation of this kind could account mainly for the enormous reduction in deaths and growth of population during the past two centuries. We must therefore consider two other possibilities: immunization and therapy; and improvements in the environment.

The contribution of immunization and therapy can be assessed by considering experience of the infections mainly responsible for the reduction of the death rate—tuberculosis, scarlet fever, measles and whooping cough. In all four, mortality had declined to a small fraction of its level in 1850 before effective medical measures were introduced. The decline of those infections in which specific measures are widely believe to have been effective—smallpox, syphilis, tetanus and possibly diphtheria—made only a small contribution to the total fall of the death rate. After a review of this and other evidence it was concluded that it was not until the twentieth century, and probably not until 1935, with the introduction of the sulphonamides that specific medical measures became available which were sufficiently powerful to reduce mortality from infection to an extent that would have influenced the national death rate.

From about 1870 there is no doubt about the contribution of one class of environmental influences, namely improvements in hygiene. Initially they comprised purification of water and sewage disposal, and their effectiveness is evident from the coincident reduction of deaths from intestinal infections.

However it is clear from changes in the death rate that the decline of mortality preceded the introduction of sanitary measures, in some countries by more than a hundred years. The most acceptable explanation is a rising standard of living, particularly improved diet which resulted from advances in agriculture.

To complete this examination of reasons for improvement in health one other influence should be mentioned, namely the limitation of numbers which followed the decline of the birth rate in the last third of the nineteenth century. It was not so much a reason for improvement in health as the means which ensured that the improvement which resulted from other influences was not lost, as previous advances in man's health were presumably lost, because of rising numbers.

In summary, the influences which were responsible for the modern improvement in health were mainly environmental (comprising two very different kinds of influences, an increase in food supplies and removal of physical hazards) and behavioural (the change in reproductive practice which restricted the growth of populations); the contribution of immunization and therapy was recent and relatively small.

However the character of medical problems has changed profoundly as a result of the decline of the infections, and it is necessary to enquire whether the major influences on health have also been transformed. The most important change is probably in the relative positions of behavioural and environmental influences. There is little doubt that until recently improvement in nutrition and protection from water and food borne disease were the more significant influences. But although these and other environmental influences are still important, in technologically advanced countries they are probably less so than the personal behaviour of the individual in relation to smoking, diet, exercise, drugs and alcohol. That is to say that in developed countries the individual's health is largely in his own hands, for by controlling his behaviour he can do more to preserve his health and extend his life than can be achieved by other preventive or therapeutic measures.

In the light of these conclusions the requirements for health can be stated simply. Those fortunate enough to be born free of significant congenital disease or disability will remain well if three basic needs are met: they must be adequately fed; they must be protected from a wide range of environmental hazards; and they must not depart radically from the pattern of personal behaviour under which man evolved, for example by smoking, overeating or sedentary living.

Changes in the character of health problems

If health planning is to be more than a series of improvisations in response to complex and changing circumstances, it should be against a background of interpretation of the predominant future health problems. While detailed prediction is impossible, there is enough information to show the main direction of current trends.

With the decline of infectious diseases, the predominant residual problems are congenital, psychiatric and geriatric. The reasons for this trend are fairly clear. The prenatal environment is difficult to investigate and control, and most diseases of children are now determined by the time of birth. Except in the case of syphilis, there is no evidence of substantial change in the frequency of the common forms of mental illness; and with the decline of infections and increased expectation of life psychiatric patients have become relatively more common. Finally, the reduction of mortality in early life and a lower birth rate have resulted in an older population in which the diseases and disabilities associated with ageing are conspicuous.

There is no more sober fact confronting health workers than the need to come to terms with these vast and relatively neglected problems. Patients with congenital, psychiatric and geriatric illnesses now occupy about two-thirds of all hospital beds and, with a rising standard of living and extension of preventive measures the proportion may well increase. In technologically advanced societies the most relevant test of the quality of medical services is no longer the work of the acute hospital, but the standard of care provided for the mentally retarded, the mentally ill and the aged sick.

The growth of technology

Another aspect of the background of health services is the spectacular and, in its financial and administrative implications, alarming advance of technology. For although future methods of investigating and treating disease cannot be foreseen, it can hardly be doubted that they will involve an enormous increase in the use, complexity and cost of technology. This development will impose its own require-ments, and will force attention to many issues, particularly in hospitals, which hitherto have been largely ignored: the small, uneconomic facility; badly located or inadequate sites; inflexible design of buildings; and lack of coordination of the services of a town or region. None of these problems is new, but the needs of technology will give them new dimensions and make it imperative to find solutions.

Against this background it can be seen that medicine is now confronted with two very different and, in some respects conflicting trends. One is towards the increased use of technology; the other is towards the predominance of patients who provide little scope for technology, but make large demands for continuing care. It is important that the framework of future services should meet and, where necessary, reconcile the requirements which arise from these trends.

To sum up: in broad terms the challenge to health services is to put due emphasis on the behavioural and environmental influences which are the main determinants of health, and within the personal medical services to seek an approach which meets and reconciles the needs of technology and care.

ISSUES IN HEALTH CARE PLANNING

Emphasis on the main influences on health

The conclusion that health is determined mainly by behavioural and environmental influences has implications for medical education and research as well as for health services. In the present context, how-ever, only the last will be considered.

In the first place, there is need for a profound change in both professional and public understanding of the determinants of health and disease. So long as it is thought that health depends primarily on personal medical care, and that diseases which are not prevented can in general be cured, there is little likelihood that sufficient attention will be given to modification of behaviour and control of the environment. For example, the public should recognize not only that cancer of the lung can be prevented, but also that little can be achieved by therapeutic measures once the disease occurs.

Secondly, it is necessary to clarify the medical role in relation to the major influences. At the present time there is some medical concern and responsibility for the general level of nutrition, reduction of smoking and control of environmental hazards. But this responsibility is less well-defined and less extensive than in the case of clinical procedures. For example, immunization against diphtheria is regarded as a medical matter in a sense that prevention of malnutrition is not, although in relation to health the latter is much the more important of the two.

In explanation of the restricted medical role it can of course be said that modification of behavioural and environmental influences is not mainly in the hands of doctors, and can be left to social workers, engineers and others. Nevertheless, there are two reasons for extension of the medical interest: first because identification of risks associated with behaviour and the environment must come largely from those concerned with disease problems; and second, because it is unlikely that sufficient attention will be given to these hazards unless they are associated in the public mind with other medical activities. It is considerations of this kind which I believe have led the Federal Department of Health and Welfare in Canada to concern itself broadly with 'Lifestyle', and to transfer responsibility for the Fitness and Amateur Sport Program from the Welfare Side to the Health Side of the Department.

Evaluation of medical procedures

It was always desirable, and with rising costs it is now essential, to assess more critically the value of clinical procedures. A distinction needs to be made between assessment of quality (which I shall define as concern with 'how well they do what they do'), effectiveness ('whether what they do is worth doing') and efficiency ('whether what they do makes better use of the resources than the available alternatives').

Assessment of quality of care is uncommon in Britain. Its acceptance will depend on education of doctors and the creation of suitable mechanisms, for example in hospitals or in association with professional bodies. It seems important to distinguish this approach to quality from investigation of efficiency (referred to below). However willing they may be to look critically at the quality of their work, individual doctors or small groups of doctors would not usually have the time, experience or interest needed to assess efficiency.

Assessment of efficiency is required not merely in preventive and therapeutic measures such as vaccines, drugs and surgery, but also in organization of care. In such assessments the randomized control is particularly, although not uniquely useful.

When a clinical procedure has been shown to be of value (i.e. 'effective'), in principle it is desirable to enquire whether it is efficient, that is whether it would make better use of the resources required than alternatives already in use or which can be introduced. This approach is particularly important if we judge that there is serious misdirection of clinical effort. There are few features of medical practice or services which would not repay investigation of this kind. Examples of subjects which may be mentioned are: the results of intervention in the various forms of congenital heart disease and the malformations of the central nervous system; the feasibility of identification of parents likely to have abnormal children (including an appraisal of genetic counselling); the contribution of amino-centesis; assessment of screening procedures; examination of hospital policies.

Decision on such issues is difficult, since many of them involve social as well as financial and medical considerations. The public is prepared to leave it to the professions to decide when the time comes to end B.C.G. vaccination, but understandably it wishes to be consulted on the choice between domiciliary and hospital obstetrics and the size and location of hospitals. Nevertheless, although such questions require value judgements which are properly matters for public and political consideration, they are also highly technical, and the value judgements cannot be made reliably without extensive professional preparation and documentation.

In the case of procedures or services already in use the difficulties of such studies, particularly of effectiveness and efficiency, are formidable. When a procedure has been adopted in clinical practice it may be considered unethical to withold it from a control population in order to assess its value. And even when a service has been shown to be of little or no value, it may be very difficult to bring it to an end after staff and facilities have been committed to it.

For these reasons I believe that evaluation should be concentrated particularly on new developments. At the present pace of technology, new procedures are likely to be more significant than those that already exist. There is a point in time when it is still possible, and ethically acceptable, to investigate the effectiveness and efficiency of a new development, before it has been introduced into medical practice. If this opportunity is unused it may not arise again.

Hospital services

In Britain there is fairly general agreement that care should be available in the community for many psychiatric, geriatric and mentally subnormal patients who are now in hospital. It is also widely accepted that hospital services should be based on a district general hospital (D.G.H.) which provides all, or nearly all, the acute services needed by the population it serves, as well as substantial psychiatric and geriatric treatment and care. There are however some differences of opinion about the size of the hospitals, their role in long term care (particularly of subnormal patients) and the need for small community hospitals for patients who do not require the full services of a D.G.H. While there are intermediate positions, the choice may be said to lie broadly between (a) a large hospital meeting all the in-patient needs of a defined population and (b) smaller hospitals which share responsibility for the services to a population.

Although the choice between these alternative approaches raises many questions, I shall refer only to the issue of principle which seems to me to lie behind it. Where services to the same population are divided between hospitals, history suggests that they become stratified into favoured (mainly acute hospitals) and depressed areas of care (psychiatric, chronic and subnormality hospitals). If this stratification continues, with the rapid advance in technology, it is likely to be even more marked than in the past. Acute hospitals, and particularly teaching hospitals, will admit patients who provide scope for technology, and the less fortunate centres will be left with responsibility for the rest, that is for the large majority. If this occurs we shall see repeated in the twenty-first century the situation described by the Webbs at the end of the nineteenth : 'The voluntary hospitals took what was interesting and the public hospitals were left with what was difficult.' The fact that all are now public hospitals will not diminish the significance of the distinction—to medical education, research and practice.

What is at issue here is a reconciliation between the needs of technology and care. Can this be achieved in the common hospital; or are there technical and psychological difficulties which make it necessary to separate them? Some people have already accepted the prospect of separation, not because they think it is desirable, but because they despair of changing the deeply rooted traditions of the hospital system.

The significance of the decision is illustrated by one of the major problems in contemporary care, namely, the care of the dying. The existing provisions within our hospitals are quite inadequate, and this has led some devoted people, motivated by strong but un-

assertive religious convictions, to establish separate units for terminal
care. But is it possible, and in another sense is it right, to expect
such institutions to carry the main responsibility for so large and
inescapable a part of the medical task?

Medical Practice

It is a remarkable feature of medical practice that while its form is
fairly uniform within a country, there are large differences in its
organization between countries. In some Australian States the
general practitioner has independent access to a hospital where he
may undertake a considerable amount of specialized work, for
example in surgery. In Britain the line between general and specialist
practice is clearly drawn; the general practitioner provides care in the
domiciliary field and refers patients needing specialist or hospital
services to a consultant. In the United States, although the pattern
varies, general practice has contracted and medical services, including
primary care, are provided largely by doctors designated as specialists.
In Israel, there are few general practitioners, and their work is
regarded by many doctors and most teachers, as an outmoded form of
medical care.

The central issue in medical practice is the relation between general
practitioner and consultant or, more broadly, between primary and
secondary care. The distinction arose during the eighteenth and nineteenth centuries when the longstanding divisions between physician,
surgeon and apothecary were replaced by a new one between doctors
with and without hospital appointments. This division has become
more significant with the increase in the amount of institutional
care and with technological developments in medicine focussed
largely on hospitals. So strong is the professional attraction of the
hospital that the question is not whether general practice can continue on traditional lines, but whether it can survive in any form.
Experience in the United States and Israel suggests that the answer
is by no means certain.

The organization of practice, like that of hospitals, should have
in view the trends and needs in technology and care. Technology
requires a high degree of specialization by medical staff, particularly
in hospital; but this must be reconciled with the needs of care,
which include primary medical care, domiciliary service and the
rehabilitation and prolonged care of the majority of hospital
patients.

These requirements may not be met without considerable changes
in medical practice affecting both general practitioner and consultant.
In some respects the issue is analogous to that discussed in relation to

hospitals: are doctors to be divided sharply into those concerned with care, including primary care, and those concerned with technology, working in hospitals? A programme under investigation in Boston assumes that a split on these lines is likely, and on the assumption that the medical graduate will be unwilling to provide primary care, proposes to explore a new type of training for health workers in this field.

As in the case of hospitals, I believe we should go to considerable lengths to avoid this stratification of technology and care. I have suggested elsewhere that the key to reorganization lies in the relation between consultants and general practitioners. 'Consultant practice should be restricted to services that require both referral and specialization as conditions of expert practice, and doctors who are not consultants should provide personal medical care in patients' homes, at a health centre and in hospital. In future it will probably be desirable for all doctors to specialize, and it is suggested tentatively that the best arrangement would be to divide the work of the personal doctor according to the age of patients. Personal medical care would then be provided by three types of doctors (paediatrician, general physician, and geriatrician) working in groups and strongly supported by consultants.'

However, it would be foolish to think that one can be confident about the ideal future organization of medical practice. Many experiments will be needed, and it is possible that different solutions will be appropriate in different circumstances (for example in urban and rural areas, and in developed and developing countries). But an essential requirement is an unrestricted evolution of the relations between practitioner and consultant and between domiciliary and hospital practice. The indispensable basis is a role for the general practitioner in hospital and a close working relation between consultant and practitioner, in and out of hospital.

Relation of doctors to other health workers

In Britain during recent years we have seen a change in the relation between doctors and social workers and between doctors and the staff of local authorities concerned with environmental health. The first change resulted from a reorganization which created a unified service under a Social Services Committee and separate from medical administration. The second change followed from the reorganization of the NHS, under which the medical specialist in environmental health transferred to the new health authorities, and retained only a consultant role in relation to local government activities in the field of environmental health.

Such changes suggest that the relation of medical to other health workers is by no means stable and may undergo further mutations. Among reasons for change are the need for rationalization, which was argued strongly in Britain in respect of social services. But there is also some dislike of what is considered to be the dominance of medical people in the health care scene, and there were undoubtedly many social environmental health workers who welcomed what they regarded as the removal of the medical yolk.

Of other fields in which the relationship may be questioned in future, much the most important is nursing. So far the nurse has accepted the fact, if not the logic, of her role. But in the United States nurses are beginning to provide primary care services which formerly would have been given by a doctor; and experiments in Britain suggest that a considerable part of the work of the general practitioner can be undertaken by the nurse to the satisfaction of the doctor and his patients.

It is possible that in time the same approach may be extended to hospitals. The fact that in past centuries the roles of apothecary and physician eventually merged suggests that there is no natural division between the tasks of prescribing for the sick and caring for the sick, and the recent medical graduate might well ask himself whether it is logical for him to prescribe the treatment to be applied by the experienced nurse who will be on the spot when the need for it arises. Some Schools in the United States have already brought the training of doctors and nurses closer together, and it is possible that in time the distinction may diminish further.

Chapter 2

THE PROVISION OF MEDICAL CARE IN HOSPITAL IN THE UNITED KINGDOM AND ITS EFFECT ON MEDICAL EDUCATION

G. A. SMART
British Postgraduate Medical Federation, London, England

BEFORE THE National Health Service came into being there were essentially three groups of hospitals in Britain—Voluntary Hospitals, which depended upon charitable gifts and upon the free services of the senior medical staff, hospitals run by local government authorities, and private nursing homes. The voluntary hospitals were charities in law and were run by a Board of Governors consisting of volunteers from the local landed gentry, from successful business men, from local authorities, trade unions, and a variety of voluntary organizations.

In general, they were the hospitals with the highest prestige. The senior staff—consultants—gave their services voluntarily, the extent of their private practices depending to a great extent on their freely given activities in the voluntary hospital. This arose from the fact that consultants only see patients referred by general practitioners or other doctors and if they did well for the 'charity' patients they tended to have proportionately more private referrals.

Almost invariably a voluntary hospital would have its own school of nursing but apart from the comparatively few large hospitals in large urban centres with associated medical schools, almost without exception they took no part in undergraduate medical education. The second group of hospitals, maintained by local government authorities, were usually, but certainly not always, of a much lower standard. They were much more often concerned with conditions of pressing concern to the public—such as infectious diseases, long-term sanatoria for tuberculosis and psychiatry. They took very little part in undergraduate education and with notable exceptions very little part in postgraduate training. Generally speaking psychiatric hospitals were institutions for the incarceration of the insane—although the word asylum denotes a haven or refuge. The medical staff, although naturally specializing in psychiatry, nevertheless were fundamentally there to attend to the physical, non-mental, illnesses of the inmates.

Private hospitals, or, as they were more often called, nursing homes, also existed in considerable numbers, although many of the voluntary hospitals had private wings. Medicine and surgery were relatively uncomplicated and most of what could be done in hospital could be done as well in nursing homes.

It should be noted that, although the oldest had been started by the teaching hospitals, for over a century all medical schools have been run by Universities and are administratively completely separate institutions from the hospitals in which clinical teaching is carried out. Very close liaison must naturally be maintained and this is usually accomplished at local level by means of a number of 'Poo-bahs' who sit on the crucial committees of both institutions. Nationally, at the present time, close liaison is maintained between the medical sub-committee of the University Grants Committee on the one hand and the Department of Health and Social Security on the other.

In 1948 the National Health Service was formed and it took over all hospitals which were not run for profit, i.e. the private nursing homes were excluded. The country was divided into a series of Regions each with a Board to administer and develop the hospital services within its Region.

However, with some exceptions each Region included—one might nearly say was centred around—that hospital which had been and was a teaching hospital by virtue of its close association with a medical school and because of the facilities it provided for teaching purposes. These hospitals, in England and Wales but not in Scotland, continued to be governed separately from the Regional Hospital Boards, each retaining its own Board of Governors which answered directly to the Ministry of Health.

Quite clearly the first task for the National Health Service in the hospital field was to upgrade the old hospitals it had inherited—particularly those which had been run by local authorities. This has taken an unconscionably long time. As my friend Henry Miller said several years ago; 'This is the only country in the world which seems to think that hospitals, like port wine, improve with age!' Nevertheless, improvement has been so great that, apart from London and one or two other of the largest towns, the proportion of hospital-type medicine done privately is very small indeed.

In April of this year the administrative structure of the National Health Service was changed so that the Regional Authorities became Regional *Health* Authorities and not just Regional *Hospital* Authorities. In other words, they are now responsible for total health care, preventive, school, and primary medical care, as well as hospital care. The teaching hospitals no longer have their own governing bodies but have become part of an Area Health Authority within a Region, and, as we shall see, this could enable changes in medical education, which were already progressively under way, to be fulfilled in a very satisfactory manner.

Having given a brief historical background, let me now turn to the traditional way in which our voluntary and hence our teaching hospitals have been organized internally, for this has had a considerable impact on medical education. The clinical services of a hospital are delivered by means of a series of teams of people called 'FIRMS'. Each 'firm' is clinically autonomous and so is each doctor of consultant or specialist rank within the firm. Typically the medical staff of a firm in a teaching hospital might consist of a consultant who is in administrative charge, and one or perhaps two other consultants who each work autonomously so far as clinical matters are concerned. These men might be whole time or part time. Patients are *their* patients and *they* are responsible for everything that happens clinically to their patients. Naturally, there may be a lot of discussion between these people about clinical problems, but no one is employed to interfere clinically in any way with another's patient. The head of the firm is head of it only in an administrative sense. Below these doctors of consultant rank there will be a number of more junior people who are either being trained in the specialty or who are spending a shorter period on the firm as part of their general postgraduate medical training. At a teaching hospital there might be a senior registrar and a registrar, perhaps a senior house officer and probably two house officers. These house officers, if the firm is a 'general' medical or 'general' surgical firm, will be occupying one of the two approved six-monthly hospital appointments which are required by law after they have graduated and before they can become legally fully registered medical practitioners.

This team of doctors will probably look after 50 or 60 beds and will in addition conduct a number of outpatient clinics each week and take their turn with the reception and care of emergencies. Such clinics are organized in various ways, but new patients, referred for an opinion by other doctors (usually general practitioners), as well as patients being followed up or reviewed are seen. Note that in accordance with previous tradition consultants do not see patients de novo except in emergency. These normally are referred by their own family doctor with a letter outlining the problem and stating any background social or family matters which might be relevant.

Traditionally most of the firms in a teaching hospital would be general medical or general surgical firms. Generally, up to about the beginning of the last war, the senior physician or senior surgeon might, although earning his living in private practice, have been appointed by the University as Professor of Medicine or of Surgery. Since that time these posts have been full-time university posts with no private practice and the clinical professors hold honorary consultant contracts with the teaching hospital (now with the Area Health Authority) and have full clinical duties and responsibilities like their consultant colleagues. They head an academic firm or unit which works strictly in parallel with the other firms. The professor does not and cannot interfere in any way with the other firms except of course in matters of teaching policy and even then what he can do in practice is very limited and depends a great deal upon his personality and relationships with his fellow consultants. The academic unit is usually more generously staffed than the other firms and at senior level there will probably be a Reader and Senior Lecturer also full-time and with honorary consultant status. Academic facilities such as research laboratories are of course also available and these will be funded by the medical school. The professor will not, nor will the other firms, carry out the routine laboratory tests for the patients on his own firm, although of course he is quite likely to carry out tests which are still in the realm of research and he may well do these at his discretion on patients throughout the hospital, but only when given permission to do so, or is requested as a favour to do so, by the consultant in charge of the patient. Routine biochemical, microbiological and pathological services are of course, like radiology, centralized as services to the whole hospital.

After two or three pre-clinical years medical students are introduced into the environment I have described. During the University term they are given a succession of systematic courses on clinical and paraclinical subjects, usually only for part of each day. Probably more than half of the clinical student's time will be spent in a series of clinical appointments and traditionally, if the firm I described had been a general medical or general surgical firm, he would have spent six months there—full-time apart from attending the lectures in the medical school. During the University vacation he would spend all his time on the firm to which he was attached. At any one time a firm might have anything from 4 to 12 students attached to it, the number depending upon the particular medical school. During this time he would generally have a series of patients allotted to him. On a medical firm he would take a full history and carry out a full physical examination. He would write this up in detail and might be expected to present the patient and all the clinical details to the consultant in charge when he was making his rounds. Naturally, the student would be 'taken over' his patients and his efforts frequently checked by the registrar or senior registrar. At one time the students' notes in some hospitals constituted part of the official case record. He would also be shown how to carry out the simpler investigative and other clinical procedures such as lumbar puncture or the aspiration of a chest. On a surgical firm he might have been expected to 'prepare' his own patients for operation—by shaving etc.—to attend and perhaps assist at the operation, and to take part in post-operative dressings and general after care. As can be seen, the traditional role of the student incorporated him with the team as someone contributing essentially to its full function. Similar appropriate activities would take place when the student was attached to firms of other disciplines such as paediatrics or gynaecology and at one time, though not now, he had to deliver a certain number of babies in the patient's own home, accompanied by a midwife.

It can be seen that up to this stage of development the hospital influence and in particular the teaching hospital influence was almost totally predominant in the clinical education of the under-graduate. However, with the continuing technical development of medicine, and with the consequent changes in the pattern of medicine as a whole and of hospital medicine in particular, the original position of apprentice occupied by the clinical medical student became in-creasingly curtailed and the way in which it was traditionally organized became more anomalous and inappropriate.

The reasons for this are not hard to find. The increased complexity of medicine enforced an ever greater degree of specialization, so that at the same time as the student needed to increase the width of his experience, the so-called general firm to which he was appointed inevitably developed its own special interests with the result that the type of clinical problems dealt with by the firm tended to be circumscribed. Increased numbers of staff, both because of increased standards and because of the rapid and essential expansion of post-graduate medical education and training, resulted in the student becoming much more of an onlooker who was 'taught at', than an active participant who learned knowledge, skills and professional attitudes by doing, with supervised professional responsibilities as a major motivating force.

Furthermore, within the hospital field some specialties such as paediatrics and psychiatry not only became as scientifically based as the fragmenting 'general' specialties, but on numerical and other grounds they were becoming of profound importance for that large proportion of students (some 40%) who would be entering general practice. Advances in medicine had themselves created new areas of importance such as geriatrics. Outside the hospital field the student was given very little first-hand experience beyond occasional visits to some of the services such as child welfare clinics run by the local authorities.

Parallel with these changes in teaching hospitals practice the regional or non-teaching hospitals have improved immensely both in the quality of the consultant staff and in their facilities. Moreover, apart from the largest hospitals which may contain specialist services for the whole region, e.g. cardiology or neurosurgery, the firms (for they are organized clinically in the same way as the teaching hospitals) have remained much more general so that anyone working there would tend to get a truer idea of the pattern of serious disease as it affects the community than he might if he were confined solely to a teaching hospital.

Moreover, in most regional hospital groups teaching centres have been developed for postgraduate and continuing education, not only of the hospital staff but also of the general practitioners or family doctors in the district. This development, which has been one of the most significant in the field of postgraduate medical education ever to have occurred in this country was given the initial support by the Nuffield Provincial Hospitals Trust and by the King Edward VII Fund which led to its enormous success. The impetus for this crystallized at a historic conference held in Oxford just eleven years ago under the auspices of the Nuffield Provincial Hospitals Trust. The facilities are generally appropriate too—or could be with very little modification—for undergraduate clinical students in rather limited numbers.

A serious fault in the medical staffing structure of our hospitals arises from the customary allocation of duties within hospital firms, which has resulted in a disproportionately large team of junior trainees relative to consultant grades of staff. In other words, really adequate junior staffing throughout the hospital service would result in too many hospital specialist trainees for the specialist or consultant vacancies which will become available. The Department of Health by agreement with the medical profession has for some years taken steps to rectify this situation by increasing the numbers of consultant posts and curtailing in oversubscribed specialties the number of trainee posts. Nevertheless we rely heavily on doctors from overseas coming to work in our hospitals to obtain postgraduate training. Many of these return to their own country and therefore do not enter into the career structure, but it should be said that in some regions of the country over 60% of the junior hospital staff have qualified overseas.

The matter has become one of controversy because the establishment of these posts is more generous in teaching hospitals and in certain parts of the country than in others, and this comparative paucity of junior staff is undoubtedly one of the main factors which would militate against the efficient training of undergraduates in more than small numbers in any given regional hospital.

Medical schools througout the country have each in their own way been attempting to come to terms with the factors I have mentioned. There is now a great deal of freedom for medical schools to experiment, for, so long as their proposals meet with the approval of the General Medical Council, they can introduce whatever changes they wish—or find possible within the stockades so readily erected by all the various vested interests within medical schools and teaching hospitals. Departmental despotism has been one of the major factors in inhibiting experiment and change in the undergraduate curriculum. Nevertheless, considerable advances *have* been made to a varying extent in different schools. These changes of course have occurred throughout the whole of the curriculum but we are here concerned only with those related to hospital practice.

As I have tried to indicate, there are six main factors which must be accommodated in these changes:— 1. The increasing complexity of hospital medicine with the consequent narrowing of interest in each clinical unit or firm (this of course extends in some instances to units combining similar medical and surgical specialties, e.g. neurology and neurosurgery). 2. The increasing disparity between the sort of conditions treated in teaching hospitals and those occurring in the community as a whole. 3. The rise in importance, because of their increasing effectiveness or of increasing social need, of subjects which in the past were only lightly dealt with. 4. The decreasing personal and responsible involvement of the student in the day to day activities of the hospital. 5. The growing importance as a discipline and specialty in its own right of domiciliary medicine with its closer connection with the behavioural sciences and community social facilities. 6. The absolute necessity for postgraduate training whatever branch of medicine is to be entered.

The general pattern of change which is emerging to cope with these problems is:— 1. To cut down the length of appointment to any one firm so that the student can experience a much wider spectrum of disciplines—including those such as family medicine which occur outside hospital. 2. To reduce or eliminate any attempt in the early clinical years to make the student an apprentice. 3. To leave less to chance and to ensure that during these early clinical years he becomes thoroughly acquainted with and has early practice in the basic clinical skills and develops attitudes which incorporates a scientific approach to solving medical problems along with a proper set of professional and humanitarian ethics. 4. To organize the curriculum and teaching so that all or most of the basic fundamentals are completed before the beginning of the final year, which can then be spent in a series of selected firms, many of which are in regional hospitals, where on the basis of his already careful training he can usefully and safely assume supervised responsibility.

Lastly, but by no means of least importance, I must mention the effect of the hospital on postgraduate education and training. It is customary in this country to divide postgraduate medical education into two segments:— 1. Professional or vocational training, which is the acquisition of experience and theoretical knowledge necessary for a particular specialty. 2. Continuing education, which really means keeping up-to-date and which is necessary throughout the whole of a doctor's active professional career.

Particularly in relation to vocational training there is an inevitable conflict between service needs on the one hand and personal educational requirements on the other. I should say at once that the Department of Health have been most imaginative and generous in this field, but quite clearly the granting of study leave, for example, must be contingent on the continuing function of the hospital services during a man's absence. Futhermore, the long hours of duty which these young people have to work hardly leaves them in a fit state to study nor indeed with much spare time in which to do it. Apart from this, considerable efforts have been made to help them.

As I have already said, most hospital groups have an academic postgraduate centre and in administrative charge of such a centre is one of the hospital senior staff who has been appointed a 'clinical tutor' by the postgraduate dean of medicine of the local university with a medical school. There are now almost 300 in the country. The postgraduate centre will have a lecture theatre, one or more rooms which can be used for seminars or for private study, a library, and audiovisual teaching aids as well as catering and other social facilities. The clinical tutor will organize lectures from visiting as well as from local people, and generally ensure that postgraduate educational activities are continually available. The social facilities are a very important factor, for here doctors of different disciplines meet, talk shop and discuss each other's problems in a purely informal way.

It is far too early yet to assess what effect the new administrative organization of the National Health Service will have on medical education. It would seem clear, however, that since the Authorities are Health and not Hospital Authorities it should become easier to utilize the whole spectrum of health care activities in the training of the student. Perhaps much more important, however, is the very great potential which lies in the development of first class and comprehensive information services so that the health needs of the population and the real impact of the health services on them can be ascertained. This knowledge must surely have a profound effect on the curriculum design and activities of medical schools, for their value to society depends very much upon their responsiveness to society's needs.

On the other hand the new organization has resulted in quite an amount of decentralization of authority. Many advantages may arise from this, but there is little doubt that it may have a potentially harmful effect on postgraduate education and training, for many of the employing authorities will simply be too small to offer all the facilities required by some of its junior trainees. Rotating training schemes have been in existence for some time and I feel sure that the new authorities would wish them to continue.

In summary, the National Health Service hospitals deal with all but a very small fraction of patients in this country who require hospitalization. This is of enormous potential advantage in the arrangements which can be made both for undergraduate clinical training and for postgraduate education. With the rapid advances of medicine and the consequent changes in priorities for health care some of the traditional disciplines may have begun to occupy too dominant a place, owing to the phase lag between community needs and educational reforms. These discrepancies are to an increasing extent being rectified and it is hoped that the new health service organization will result in effective information services which will tend to keep education and training more closely in line with requirements.

Chapter 3

THE PROVISION OF MEDICAL CARE IN THE COMMUNITY

G. K. H. Hodgkin
Memorial University, St John's, Newfoundland, Canada

MY OWN personal experience of helth care delivery has been of three different kinds viz. Private practice in Britain for 5 years (1949–54); National Health Service practice in Britain for 20 years (1954–73); and Medicare practice in Canada for 18 months (1973–74) with item-of-service payment by Medicare.

I speak not as an academic nor as an administrator but as a working general practitioner—one of the 'pawns' whom the administrators have to utilize, assist and sometimes manipulate. I want to speak from my personal 'coal-face' experience of the three systems of health care delivery because they represent almost the total spectrum of methods used by different countries in the western world. I should say that at all times I have enjoyed this 'coal-face' experience enormously, despite its difficulties and occasional frustrations.

First, I wish to introduce the concept of the Dilemma of Service, which will then enable me to analyse, compare and contrast my personal experience of these three different systems. Secondly, by analysing my own experience I hope to demonstrate my reasons for drawing two basic conclusions about health care delivery; namely, that doctors are idealistically as well as financially motivated, therefore it is essential that in any health care delivery system methods of payment should *reinforce* and *not conflict* with such idealism; and that the 'dilemma of service' requires that every community as it becomes organized will ultimately demand a health care service in which doctors are paid by a flexible combination of different methods which take into account the conflicting demands of the dilemma of service.

The Dilemma of Service

The best illustration of this is taken from the world of business. Figure 1 represents the management grid (*Ref.* Blake & Moulton, *Gulf Press* 1964). This is a graphic representation of the two conflicting elements of the dilemma that affects anyone who is providing any form of service. It illustrates the degrees of concern for the needs of the individual (10 arbitrary degrees) and the degree

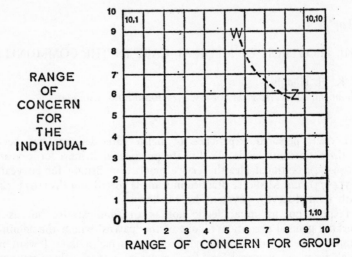

Fig. 1. The Management Grid

of concern for the needs of the group or wider community (10 arbitrary degrees).

The same dilemma affects teachers, lawyers, shopkeepers and all public servants, but nowhere is it better demonstrated than in the world of modern medicine. The management grid allows any service to be plotted according to these two elements in a way that allows a degree of generalization about the services provided. Thus a 10,1 practice at A will provide a very high standard of personal service to relatively few individuals. This service will tend to have the following characteristics:

Advantages:
    A very personal service to the patient.
    Excellent utilization of every complex technical procedure with little regard to cost, either in terms of manpower or finance.
    High patient satisfaction.
    High job satisfaction for the doctor.
Disadvantages:
    A poor or very patchy delivery of the service to the total community. Doctors will find it difficult to extend their individualized service from the privileged few to the rest of the community. Shortages of money and doctors combined with simple difficulties of distance may prevent its wider application to the whole community.

The actual practice of this kind of personalized medicine often blinds the profession to the severe and often extreme needs of the rest of the community.

The doctors find it hard to delegate and may even try to be a 'maid of all work' i.e. type letters, remove gall bladders, set fractures or be a specialist who spends his time doing general practice.

Private practice, hospital medicine and any item of service-based insurance all tend to provide this kind of service.

At the other extreme of the dilemma is the 1,10 practice (at point B). This aims to deliver medical care to the whole community, but in so doing loses its personal element.

Advantages:

Deals effectively with large quantities of patients.

Community priorities are usually clearly defined and all sections of the community receive the same standard of service.

Dependence of the patient on the doctor is discouraged.

Delegation of the doctors' responsibilities may lead to a wide ranging service. Thus widespread preventative measures such as total measles prophylaxis are encouraged because a nurse can carry them out and because they ultimately save the doctor's time.

Many traditional medical responsibilities can be delegated to specially trained non-medical staff e.g. normal midwifery, cardiographs and minor surgery.

Disadvantages:

Individual patients are less well satisfied because the service may be impersonal.

Patients easily feel neglected because personal or emotional problems are easily overlooked.

Job satisfaction for doctors can be low.

Information flow within the necessarily large organization may be inhibited or distorted.

Polyclinic practice, some large urban practices in Britain and practices in underdeveloped countries are examples of this type of service.

The ideal between these two extremes is the 10,10 practice at point C which aims despite shortages of doctors and limited resources to deliver a personalized service to the whole community. This is the unattainable goal that every primary physician must continually strive for. There are two practical methods of moving towards this ideal in that the doctor can prune or modify unnecessary or time-consuming procedures—the work-study approach; and he can delegate i.e. transfer to a less well paid helper any job that can be done as well (or better) by someone other than the doctor.

If the doctor is to utilize either or both of these methods a very important principle is involved: *'The doctor (and the community) not the patient must decide priorities.'* This is one of the basic reasons why any system which involves direct payment of the doctor by the patient tends inevitably to be associated with a poor overall delivery of health care. If a patient is used to paying a doctor twenty dollars to have his ears syringed, it is difficult for the doctor to delegate this procedure to a nurse, because the patient is likely to be upset.

Influences affecting the 'Dilemma of Service'

I propose to discuss the five main factors that have influenced me in my role as a primary physician working at the 'coal-face' under various systems of health care delivery.

1. The reverse correlation of health with wealth.
2. The 'iceberg' of unreported morbidity.
3. The wide variation in the demand and needs of different communities.
4. The Hospitals orientation of modern medicine.
5. Methods of payment.

1. *The reverse correlation of ill health with wealth*

This reverse correlation applies to communities as a whole as well as individuals. Thus the poorer any community is, the greater the morbidity and the higher the mortality rate; also in any individual's life his medical needs are greatest when he is earning least i.e. in youth, in old age and when sickness prevents him earning.

I found the effect of moving from private practice to NHS practice very dramatic in this context. To know that you can utilize any effective treatment, however costly, for the benefit of even the poorest patient is a boon that I only fully realized after entering the service. To see patients as often as I like without being suspected of hidden financial motives greatly benefitted the doctor-patient relationships.

This reverse correlation in all those communities in which I have worked appeared to have created a drive by each community to move away from individual payment of doctors by patients, towards some system of insurance and ultimately to both compulsory as well as comprehensive insurance; whether this was called 'socialized medicine', medicare, etc., appeared to matter very little.

The demand for a compulsory system has its roots in the reverse correlation of wealth and lack of patient foresight; thus lack is also correlated with poverty, rendering compulsory insurance necessary. Similarly, if an insurance is not comprehensive, many anomalies arise, e.g. in Canadian medicare practice, drugs are free in hospital but are paid for outside—I find it is not uncommon for a child of poor parents to be brought to me (a G.P.) for treatment of an acute respiratory infection; on discovering the cost of the drugs the parents take the child to the hospital emergency department, where needless dual care is paid for by the community.

Similar examples are plentiful, perhaps the most striking occurs in the United States, where many patients are admitted to hospital for Blue Cross treatment of conditions that could have been handled more efficiently in the community, but for which Blue Cross payments are not available.

Thus we begin to see the developed Western communities bringing pressure to bear on doctors to move away from the 10,1 position (fig. 1) of private practice towards the 1,10 or 10,10 positions that require some form of comprehensive medical insurance.

2. The 'iceberg' of unreported morbidity

If all patients reported every symptom or complaint to the doctor it has been estimated that doctor/patient contacts would increase fourfold. The doctor is in a dilemma, if he discourages patients from reporting illness, it is frequently those patients who most need the doctor that are discouraged. If he is to diagnose disease in its early stages he must always encourage the reporting of morbidity; if the patient could decide himself what is serious and what is trivial the primary physician would have little justification for his existence. If the primary physician is to encourage patients to report—as clearly he should—then there appears to be only one effective solution and this is some form of initial screening process that involves paramedical staff.

The effects of the 'iceberg'

The iceberg has considerable clinical effects, thus it is much harder to pick out the one case of cough or headache that is caused by serious disease, if this is encountered amongst a hundred other cases of trivial origin. Apart from this the iceberg has a tremendous impact on systems of health care delivery:

If doctors are paid by the patient direct, poor patients tend to report serious disease too late for effective treatment.

If doctors are paid by the community on a full time basis or by capitation, the doctors are easily overwhelmed, because the financial barriers to reporting morbidity are removed. This happened in the early days of the NHS until financial incentives to delegate work load were introduced.

If doctors are paid by the community, on an item-of-service basis, the iceberg and the undifferentiated nature of primary care are so large that the community soon becomes unable to pay doctors to deal with this on their own and pressure is brought on doctors to delegate. The financial incentives inevitably drive the doctors to uncover increasing quantities of unreported morbidity.

3. *The wider variations in the demands and needs of different communities*

When I went to Newfoundland I had never removed a tooth in my life, but in St John's dental care must be paid for and there is a shortage of dentists. I now find myself removing teeth. Similarly a friend of mine in Basutoland reached an amicable agreement with a witch doctor; he agreed to refer all his social and psychological problems to the local medicine men, provided the latter referred all painful or obviously physical problems to my friend. He said this was an excellent arrangement, because in fact in this situation my friend lacked the staff and the understanding required to deal with much of the social and psychological work.

The hospital achieves its amazing diagnostic and therapeutic successes because the doctor can control almost completely the environment of the patient. In the community the primary physician treats the patient in an uncontrolled environment. Thus one of the main jobs of the primary physician is to act as a nodal 'triage' point between uncontrolled (community) and fixed (hospital) environments.

The effects of the varying needs of different communities

As we have seen in the two extreme examples given above, solution of this problem has three aspects; viz. acquisition of new skills, a flexible approach, and a preparedness to delegate to others. The best solution to this problem of varying needs is for each medical school to relate its primary care needs to the community of which it is a centre. This concept inevitably conflicts somewhat with the desire of all medical schools to produce a basic undifferentiated doctor.

Methods of payment however also affect both the flexibility of the doctor and his preparedness to delegate. Thus in a capitation or full-time service, there is a tendency for primary physicians to delegate too much to specialists, nursing staff or social workers, whereas in insurance or private practices which are based on items of service it is very difficult to persuade doctors to delegate at all.

It seems that if we are to approach the 10,10 position (fig. 1) we may have to combine the benefits of paying doctors on an item-of-service and a full-time basis.

4. The hospital orientation of modern medicine

Most medical schools are built round a hospital training and there is no doubt that this is an excellent method of training. But hospital is essentially an individual 10,1 type of medicine, and it is important therefore to introduce early to medical students an awareness of the need in every doctor to consider the needs of the community as well as those of each individual. The introduction of the general practitioner to undergraduate training allows this to be done in a way that makes sense to medical students. The general practitioner provides a 'role model' of the clinician who really every day faces the dilemma of service.

5. Methods of payment

Doctors are idealistically as well as financially motivated and it is vital therefore to introduce a system of payment that reinforces without conflicting with their idealism. If the dilemma of service is to be solved then a dual flexible method of payment would seem vital, i.e. one which encourages doctors to service the needs of both the individual and the community. In effect, this is happening in both Britain and Canada, despite their essentially opposite original approach.

Once private practice has been recognized as an inefficient form of health care delivery we find that Canada is having to modify its item-of-service insurance payments to encompass incentives that improve the service to the community as a whole, while Britain has had to modify her capitation or full-time service payments to include item-of-service loadings for old people and others.

The conclusion is clear : a dual system of payment is essential if the ideal (10,10) service is to be provided for our patients in which item-of-service elements and capitation or fixed salary are both present and can be varied according to the needs of the community and the resources (doctors, money, etc.) available.

Chapter 4

HEALTH CARE IN THE FEDERAL REPUBLIC OF GERMANY
AND ITS EFFECT ON EDUCATION, SPECIALISATION AND
SETTLEMENT OF DOCTORS

W. D. GERMER
Innere Abteilung Städtische Wenckebach-Krankenhaus, Berlin-Tempelhof

HISTORICALLY THE German social legislation dates back to the year 1883 when the law of sickness insurance was first proclaimed. Then followed the respective laws of compensation for industrial injuries and other professionally acquired diseases in 1884 and that of old-age and invalidity insurance in 1889. Finally in 1911 these laws were put together in the so called insurance decree of the Reich and supplemented by a decree of survivor insurance.

There are both voluntary and compulsory insurances in Germany. 99,1% of all Germans are insured against sickness either way. More than 90% of the population belong to the legal sickness insurance, a total of 32,8 million persons being direct members of the legal sick-insurance-funds for instance the local-, the works- the guild- and the compensation-sick-funds. In addition to that the relatives of the direct members are also insured bringing the total of legally insured persons up to 55,8 millions.

The income limit for compulsory sickness insurance in the Federal Republic of Germany of today lies with DM 22.500 a year. Costs for these funds are shared by employer and employee respectively worker equivalently. In case of sickness, pregnancy or death all costs either ambulatory or hospital costs including maternity help and burial money are covered by the insurance. Since 1970 a law of continued payment of wages for the sick is in force.

The recent unusually high-rising rates of the expenditures of the legal sick-funds in Germany, which exceeds by far the general inflation, have to be looked at against the background of a variety of developments.

1. The efficiency catalogue of these funds has permanently been broadened including recently measures for the early detection of diseases like disorders of development in infancy and genital cancers of both sexes.
2. The medical offer has definitively been improved through

more doctors, more hospital beds, better instruments and apparatus for diagnosis and therapy, more effective drugs and new arrangements for both preventive care and rehabilitation.

3. There is a growing consciousness for health matters in the German population which claims for a qualitative- and quantitatively better and therefore more expensive health care.

4. The number of old people over 65 years of age who require the health services especially, is rising both absolutely and proportionally measured to the total population from scarcely 13% in 1968 to about 14,5% in 1974.

Table I

Membership of Legal Sickness Insurance

Year	Members	Aged or Disabled	% of Aged or Disabled
1960	21,556,514	5,503,528	20%
1965	22,855,578	5,884,187	20%
1972	23,800,605	9,023,496	28%

Table 1 illustrates for 3 different years the relation of active membership and old aged and disabled persons belonging to the German funds of legal sickness insurance. The percentage of annuitants has risen in 7 years at 8%.

Table II

Hospital Beds in W. Germany 1972

3,519 Hospitals   700,263 Beds

9.8 Mill. People treated	Average stay in H. = 23.9d.
Public H. = 54%	Pro 10,000 Inhab. = 114be.
Free P. Utility H. = 36%	20% internal Wards
Private H. = 10%	19% surgical Wards
Hospitals: > 1000 beds = 2.5%	Hospital Personnel = 611,700

At the end of 1972 there were 700.263 beds available in 3.519 hospitals in the Federal Republic of Germany. In these beds 9.8 Million hospital patients were treated in that year. The average stay of a patient in hospital amounted to 23.9 days, the average degree of utilisation of a hospital thus being 87%.

With 114 beds pro 10.000 inhabitants a new maximum has been reached. 54% of the beds are to be found in public, 36% in free public utility and 10% only in private hospitals. The prevailing disciplines are internal medicine with 20% and surgery with 19% of these beds. The trend to the big hospital continues. Big hospitals with more than 1.000 beds represent indeed only 2,5%, they comprise however 19% of the total bed offer of the German hospitals.

Definitively more than the number of hospital beds increased the number of hospital personnel which totaled at the end of 1973 611.700 persons.

Table III

Hospital Bed Per Inhabitant, Doctor and Nurse

Year	Inhabitant per bed	Doctor per bed	Nurse per bed
1960	96	18.9	5.3
1968	91	17.1	4.4
1972	86	13.3	3.4

Whereas a hospital doctor in 1960 had to care for 18,9 beds in 1972 there were 13,3 beds only to be cared for by him, and whereas a hospital nurse had to service 5,3 beds in 1960, there were only 3,4 beds pro nurse in 1972.

Accordingly with the salaries of the hospital personnel having risen substantially during these years it is small wonder that more than 80% of the total expenditures of the German hospitals is used up for the payment of wages both for nursing personnel and doctors.

Table IV

Active Doctors and Med. Assistants in W. Germany

Year	Doctors total	Female Doctors	Inhabitants per Doc.	Med. Assistants	Female Med. A.
1960	79,350	12,538	703	3328	599
1965	85,801	14,739	691	6613	2001
1972	103,910	20,192	592 (340–708)	5445	1281

The number of doctors and of medical assistants increased in West Germany during the years 1960–1972 at an average yearly rate of 2,5%. There were 32% more educated medical people in 1972 than there were 12 years ago in 1960. The table illustrates also both the female portion of doctors amounting in 1972 to 1/5 of the total- and the ratio: inhabitant/doctor for the 3 cited years, the latter being 592 inhabitants pro doctor in 1972 with a fluctuation from 340–708.

Table V

Health Service Personnel In W. Germany 1972

Doctors {	In Free Practice	(1960: 49,225)–51,159
	In Hospitals	(1960: 22,646)–42,245
	Administration and Research	(1960: 7479)–10,506
Med. Assistants		5445
Pharmacists		22,551
Dentists		31,405
Nurses		212,296

In 1972 out of the total number 51.159 doctors compared with 42.245 in 1960 were working in free practice in distinct contrast to that 42.245 against only 22.646 doctors worked full time in hospitals. 10.506 doctors of the total sum compared to 7.479, 12 years ago worked in either administration or research.

This remarkable numerical shift from the doctor working in free practice to the doctor working in hospital is a rather recent event in our country the reasons for which being manifold. The methods and means of modern medicine which have been refined and specialized to such a high degree in recent years on one hand and the less strenous working conditions in a team as compared with a one man practice on the other are undoubtedly important motives for this movement.

In this connection it is important to mention that the separation between treatment of a patient in free practice and of a patient in hospital is in Germany a very definite one in so far as only the University clinics are doing ambulatory work, in their polyclinics and neither practitioner nor specialist from outside has any professional duty or influence upon the in patients, the post of a consultant for such a person being the rare exception.

There are recently strong tendencies to alter this situation and to equip the public hospitals or at least the recently established teaching hospitals with ambulatory services, tendencies which have the support of both the influential trade unions and the sick-insurance funds. So far the union of the German panel-doctors is however opposed to the idea of opening polyclinics in public hospitals referring to the very good supply with medical care of the German population for the time being by the doctors in free practice.

And indeed the Federal Republic of Germany has in comparison with other European countries a rather high average density of physicians. The problem of securing and guaranteeing the ambulatory medical care by—in 1973—some 55.600 panel-doctors lies however primarily in the uneven geographical distribution of the doctors in both urban, fringe and rural areas and their uneven distribution in the different medical disciplines.

Whereas the average relation of panel-doctor to legally insured people lies around 1 : 1.000 insured persons in the whole of Western Germany this situation is very different in rural areas or urban fringe areas where the ratio doctor to inhabitant may be 1 : 2.700 or in case of a specialist even 1 : 5.000 or more.

The union of the German panel-doctors is trying to change this state of affairs by a variety of mainly financial impulses and facilitations like guarantees of revenues, loans without interests, arrangements of central or partial practice communities, allowances to engage assistants etc. Unfortunately the response to all these endeavours is not too good. 'Urbanisation' of the doctors is probably going to continue in Germany unless the State does not interfere. There are political forces today which aspire to a prohibition of the free settlement of a panel-doctor in a place he prefers whenever unfavourable places are still medically uncovered.

On the other hand it is since some years impossible to fill the medical posts in both the public health- and in the medical army-services.

This picture of the situation of the German doctor would not be complete without mentioning the foreign doctors working in Germany today. Among the 111,721 doctors working in Germany in 1974 there were 5.808 or 5,3% foreigners prevailingly Iranians (19%), Turks (10,9%) and Yugoslavs (9,9%). Since these foreign doctors mainly work in clinics and hospitals they represent, in some rural hospitals between 20-30% of the total medical staff.

The system of medical education has experienced great changes in recent years in West-Germany. The new order of medical graduation, the so called approbation, is coming into full operation—to be sure—only from 1975 onwards. The last year of study at the medical schools is going to be changed into a practical-internship-year thereby shortening the length of the medical study to 5 years. That means inter alia that in order to avoid overcrowding of the medical schools by students looking for practical instruction many urban hospitals have to be turned into teaching hospitals in the very near future. Since such teaching hospitals do not exist at all in Germany at the moment this will be no small task.

The reforms already started in the schools where the last 3 years of attendance are much more directed now towards the later professional activities than before and more subjects of choice have been introduced already. In August of this year a uniform, written preliminary medical examination, the so called Physikum, has been held for the first time in the whole Federal Republic in form of a quiz. It is to be hoped that the judgment of the students becomes more just by this procedure than by the individual examination so far.

There is a numerus clausus at all German medical schools at the moment the applicants being choosen by the addition of their marks at the final examinations in school. This rather crude method of selection is going to be replaced shortly by the employment of neutral interviewers by the Universities.

Also the German medical curriculum has experienced important changes recently. The new curriculum emphasizes especially the importance of subjects like social medicine, labour medicine, psycho-somatic medicine, family planning and preventive medicine.

In conclusion I would like to mention still very briefly some problems of postgraduate training in the Federal Republic. There exists of course a very widely famed offer of possibilities to continue one's studies in medicine after graduation reaching from the monthly meetings of the small district club of doctors over seminars, symposia and other forms of lectures arranged by both the regional or federal Chamber of physicians, by medical unions, by pharmaceutical firms and other bodies to the big congresses devoted to either some medical speciality or to laboratory diagnosis, to therapy or to an assortment of themes.

Since a certain percentage of doctors always does however not participate in any form of postgraduate training, tendencies have recently been voiced to make this training obligatory and to check the results by repeated examinations. Likewise one intends to introduce formal examinations before bestowing upon some one the degree of a specialist in a medical discipline. This has until now been done in Germany by the medical Chambers upon proposal and recommendation of the superior of the one concerned. So in all the fields of health I tried to touch upon in this paper the State is gaining ground. If to a better future I do not dare to prophesy.

Chapter 5

THE PROVISION OF MEDICAL CARE IN GERMAN HOSPITALS AND ITS EFFECT ON EDUCATION

E. SEIDLER
Albert-Ludwigs-Universität, Freiburg, Germany

ONE CAN assume that at this publication, in which representatives of many countries participate, every country tends to present its best side to the subject of medical care. Therefore, at the beginning of my topic, I would like to apologize for the complex situation in West Germany, which forces me to characterize the present problems of the hospital and of medical education in a critical way. Certainly, I do not want, as we say in Germany, to dirty our own nest; however, I would like to touch on a few fundamental problems of medical care which I believe go beyond the borders of West Germany. Therefore I have divided my contribution into four parts:

First, I want to introduce my topic with a few spotlights on problems of tradition. I think there is almost no field where such strong traditional structures so impressively confront actual demands.

After this I will discuss the present situation in Germany, then the tendencies in hospital development, and in conclusion I have to speak on the relationship between hospital and medical education.

In West Germany the number of publications and suggestions to reform and to improve the hospital situation are uncountable. All of them have in common the complaint that the patient who seeks and who needs help is in danger of being sacrificed to the administrative demands of the institution. The reasons for this are contained in numerous factors, most of which can be understood as the burden of non-reflected traditional elements.

The hospital can be classified according to three social-functional demands: general cultural; personal institutional; and individual. First, the hospital serves the whole society as a place for people who need to be taken care of; this in a more increasing degree as the relationship of subjective need and objective help is transferred from the group to the institution. The second function states that no institution can be regarded as an isolated unit; therefore, the hospital must be recognized as representing other institutions: the state, the sciences, the economy, the family, the school, etc. The third function, the private function of the hospital, has a double aspect. On the one hand the individual expects an optimal offer of diagnostic, therapeutic and nursing possibilities. On the other hand the institution itself must guarantee the fulfillment of this task; specifically through the teamwork of the people working in the hospital.

All of these functions, in the external structure as well as in the world of the patients and of their caretakers, are strongly formed by traditional schemes. The principle of relieving society of people who need to be cared for is the oldest motif in hospital tradition. As long as the conception of the old traditional hospital was of a refuge for all social, physical, and psychical frailty, the institution bore the character of a social asylum. Illness was therefore only one among many possible forms of indigence, sharing with those forms the aspect of poverty. The hospital acquired the double character of the refuge and of the socially-ordered institution. Therefore, in the case of the socially disturbing illnesses (communicable diseases, psychic disorders), the basic motif of the traditional hospital has been determined by social morals not by medical science. Social morals also determined the function and the behavior of the hospital staff. At best, medicine in the traditional hospital played a consulting role, whereas most of the care must be understood as nursing care.

In a narrow sense it can be said that the idea of the modern hospital dates only back to the eighteenth century when institutions were built only for the purpose of admitting sick people and with the aims of treating patients and winning medical knowledge. All other social illnesses were referred to other institutions, the interest of the public having shifted from care to cure and, therefore, to a shorted stay in the hospital. Because of this the hospital entered at the beginning of the nineteenth century a crisis of structure and organization which, I believe, still continues today. This crisis can be characterized by the following points:

a. Medicine has established itself in the hospital as a dominating and purposive role carrier. The successful experience of the method of natural sciences in medicine seemingly established the hospital as a place for the unlimited winning and application of knowledge. Optimal medical care is equated with differentiated fields of specialization, with highly refined instruments, and with various technical functions working together flawlessly.

b. Nursing, with its task of satisfying basic human needs, becomes less a part of the therapeutic plan than of the carrying-out of medical instructions. This is supported by the development of a heterogenous self-understanding of nursing as a particular organization with hard to overcome tendency to regard itself separately and clearly from the medical profession.

c. The management of the hospital falls increasingly into the category of the industrial management of a large enterprise, especially since, with the growing agglomeration of population centers, the trend towards large hospitals has become common.

d. The ascent of medicine in the nineteenth century moved medicine into the center of governmentally planned politics. As an important factor in social politics, the hospital received the task of fighting and preventing illnesses in order to lower the death rate and subsequently to raise the level of public health. The highest principle of hospital care became the restoration of efficiency.

e. For the patient in the hospital these developments had serious and lasting consequences. The scientific medicine mainly saw him as the organic patient; as his personal suffering became impersonalized he became a case. The increasingly larger and more technically complicated hospital saw him as a numerical factor which had to be classified, administered, and discharged. The form of patient hospitalization, as well as building structure and administrative technique, had to orientate on economic management; the problems of living space, the lease of life, and the need for rest, basically contradicted the aim of the hospital. There arose towards the hospital that deep ambivalence between anxiety and trust which we have to account for in all of our problems, problems for which various motives—historical and actual, scientific and social, public and private—are responsible.

The present situation

It is absolutely necessary to keep all of these developmental factors in mind, if one is to be aware of the present situation in hospital care. In a law passed in West Germany in 1972 to finance hospitals, hospitals are defined as 'institutions in which illnesses, complaints, or bodily injuries are diagnosed, cured, or eased by medical and nursing help; and in which child delivery is performed and the persons requiring treatment accommodated and cared for.' Certainly such a legal definition wants to create the possibility of influencing the interior and exterior structure of the hospital on a political level; yet the legal definition points out very clearly the problems of the hospital as a social institution. In fact the hospital also has a central meaning in the social structure of West Germany which can be proved by the following striking figures:

One out of every forty-two employees in West Germany works in a hospital; in 1971, 520,000 people were employed in this field. Between 1960 and 1968 the total number of hospitalized patients increased more than 20%. In a community of 10,000 people, the increase amounts to an additional 2,000 hospitalized yearly. In the same period of time the number of births in the hospital increased from 66.2% of the total births in the community to 91.6%; also, deaths in the hospital increased from 43.9% of the total deaths in the community to 51.5%. This means nearly every child is born in the hospital and that every second person dies there. In 1971 the Statistical Yearbook listed 3,545 hospitals in West Germany totalling approximately 700,000 beds, 213,000 non-medical staff, and 104,000 doctors. 55% of the available beds were financed by the public, in contrast to 36% by charitable contributions and 9% by private individuals.

These latter three characteristics show the legal situation of hospitals in our country. The greatest part is financed by the public; this means by local, state, and to a small degree, federal government. The thirty-seven percent of the so-called charitable hospitals are very strongly influenced by religious societies: parishes, religious orders, and charitable institutions, all of whose properties are earmarked. Not earmarked and, therefore available for other purposes, are properties invested in the so-called private hospitals. Supporters of those hospitals are mainly doctors. Although their contribution to the total number of hospital beds is small, it is increasing remarkably.

The figures mentioned do not show the increasing structural crisis of the hospitals. Regarded totally, the hospital succeeds only with great difficulty in satisfying its organizational, legal, and financial needs. Presently the yearly gross earnings of hospitals total twenty milliards DM, a figure which corresponds to the gross earnings of the postal service or of the railroad. The total yearly cost deficit is also high, now estimated at over 2 milliards DM per year. Hospitalization fees do not cover costs, and rapidly increasing staff and equipment costs intensify the problem; the law to finance hospitals attempts to change these things; however, it has not yet been very effective. In addition, in spite of the destruction of the Second World War, 35% of all hospitals in Germany are more than fifty years old, and the plans for new buildings still can not keep pace with immensely increasing needs.

These are exterior circumstances: now we should view the interior structure of the German hospital. Hospitals are functionally distinguished by an official definition as being either special hospitals (Sonderkrankenhäuser) or acute hospitals (Akutkrankenhäuser). Acute hospitals can be understood as hospitals which treat patients who normally regain their health after a short period of time. In this class belong the so-called general hospitals which combine several medical specialities under one management, and hospitalize patients regardless of their age or type of illness. Also classed with the acute hospitals are the so-called special hospitals (Fachkrankenhäuser) which only admit patients who suffer from certain specific illnesses or of a certain age group. Some of these hospitals restrict themselves to specific types of medical treatment. In contrast, special hospitals are hospitals for illness and rehabilitation requiring lengthy treatment.

Independent of the definitions just given, German hospitals show a typical organizational and functional structure which can be defined on a horizontal and vertical plane. The horizontal structure is determined by three areas of different operational function: the medical function (diagnosis, therapy), the nursing function (direct and indirect nursing care, auxiliary medical services), and the administrative and economic function (management, maintenance). All three areas are directly controlled by the hospital director, who is the legal representative for the owner of the hospital.

The vertical structure implies both the organizational executive framework of the hospital, and its authority structure. At the top are the medical director, the superior nurse, and the administrative director, all of whom have to make basic decisions and to assume responsibilities for these decisions.

This classical model is the source of numerous conflict situations which at this time abound in German hospitals. In the previous years several suggestions have been made to reform this structure. I would like to show you only a few of these models. The most popular hospital plan is the so-called classless hospital. Its purpose is to overcome the old division of the hospital into nursing classes, to introduce into the hospital a democratic structure of organization and leadership, to abolish the private liquidation rights of head doctors, and to equalize nursing fees. The department model, on the other hand, tries to achieve a better hospital structure by making the departments smaller by increasing the number of medical specialities in the hospital. Here also one endeavors to abolish traditional hierarchical forms of organization, and above all to achieve, through the unification of conservative, operational, and theoretical departments of the hospital, medical centers which provide patients with expert medical care. There are other models—from the German hospital community, from doctors, from universities, from doctors, from private communities—all of which seem more to reflect specific group interests than to provide basic analytic ideas. To loosen the rigid borders of the acute and special hospitals, it has also been suggested in Germany that the different types of hospitals be unified in a 'balanced hospital community'.

Tendencies in hospital development

There is no doubt that, from individual behaviour to local structure, the hospital of today is bound more to the principles of yesterday than such analytically justified changes would suggest. The trends of hospital development today are directed mainly towards the sole improvement in efficiency, except in the single cases where there is an idea of a new structuring the total health system. Therefore, most of the reform ideas are still directed towards healing the patient faster and better. As a sole planning goal, this fails. Already under the present system of public health, the problems of ambulatory and non-ambulatory patients, of chronically and acutely ill patients, and the demands of prophylaxis, of early diagnosis, of rehabilitation, and of social medicine, focus so much attention on the medicine of the hospital that a one-dimensional planning geared only to the problem of healing diseases can no longer master the total task of the hospital.

These and other suggestions for reform must face the fact that the demands upon the institution of the hospital are basically changing. Not only will medical achievements of an unknown nature shortly take place in the hospital; but also, with the trend towards a shortened work period and increased life span, every human being will not only be born and die in the hospital, but will also spend an increasing part of his existence there. Therefore, both the treatment of acute illness and the recovery represent only one aspect of the hospital. Perhaps the conception of the hospital of the future has to begin at that point from which the basic idea of the hospital started: with the assurance of exterior and interior living space for frailty of all kinds.

The relationship between hospital and medical education

Concerning medical education in such structured hospitals in West Germany, one must add some basic ideas. Since medieval times, medicine in Germany was an ordinary part of university faculties. Although medicine then was only a field of bookish erudition (the hospital, too, rarely educated students practically), as it was almost everywhere, the strong unity in the university significantly determined the medical training. This pertains also both to the structure of the medical faculty and to the basic method of medical teaching. It was, and it remains, a characteristic of the German medical education that it is principally based on imparting theoretical knowledge to which the practical aspect of medical training is added. Until now, therefore, a clear distinction between theory and practice was made, theory being taught by institutions of which most had little or no connection with the university hospitals.

University hospitals likewise show a specific structure. These clinics were conceived in the middle of the nineteenth century with the idea of assuring simultaneously the tasks of teaching, research, and the care of people. This still has today the consequence that doctors working in those hospitals must fulfill all three tasks. Because until recently only university hospitals were authorized to teach medicine, all other hospitals, for example municipal hospitals, had no role in the education process. Moreover, the university hospital staff must perform clinical research using its own equipment; this in addition to its chief daily task of caring for people.

Therefore, we have in Germany a faculty structure which is divided into a theoretical and clinical part; the equivalent teaching institutions, the institutes and the hospitals, have traditionally adapted this structure. Until three years ago medical education was similarly divided. At earliest, the medical student saw the inside of a hospital in his third year of education, after he had completed the so-called pre-medical education by passing his pre-medical examination (Physikum) and began the clinical part of his studies. These clinical studies took place mainly in the hospital and consisted chiefly of demonstration lectures, and courses on the learning of technical skills. Up to the final exam, practical experience with the patients was minimal; therefore, the license to practice medicine depended on practical time spent in the hospital after the exam.

It is our current and singular problem in Germany, that for three years now a new educational model has been legalized which must be realized within the framework of the old existing institutions. It is clear that an institution such as the hospital, in all its elements, is bound to past structures, and that we are therefore in Germany in an evolutionary period which does not permit me to reply properly to the topic; moreover, all the present, acute difficulties hinder the possibility of describing the new relationship between hospital and medical training.

I do not have to talk about the long and painful process which led to the new way of education. For the present topic it is important to note that four steps mark the way of the present education, namely, a shorter pre-clinical part, a clinical-theoretical part, a clinical-practical part, and one year of practical work in the required clinical subjects. With this change it is evident that hospitals are now much more involved in medical studies; on the other hand, it is also evident that our problems have only just begun.

These problems are on two levels. First, it is impressing that the new way of education is shorter and more compressed. With this planning it was overlooked that the shorter and more compressed medical training necessitates a basic re-thinking of the curriculum. The separate disciplines have been asked to unify their teaching materials in so-called catalogues of learning aims, especially with respect to the new written examination. These catalogues, still in the experimental stage, are not yet satisfactory; specifically, they contain so much informational material that the student is now forced to learn more in a shorter period of time.

It has to be emphasized that the new educational structure demands a greater adherence to practice, for example, instruction in smaller groups with numerous lessons at the sickbed. But this confronts us with a second problem : our institutes and our hospitals are, in their constructional conception and in their interior structure, planned after the old educational system. Without sufficient planning, without sufficient financial aid, and without an enlargement of buildings, faculties do not feel capable of realizing a medical education which is close to practice. There are not enough teachers for teaching in smaller groups. The number of beds and the general capacity for patients in the hospital still limit the number of students. Therefore, the hospital is the bottleneck in the medical education which causes one of our biggest problems, namely the increasing restriction in admissions to medical education.

Because the structure and the capacity of the hospital no longer met all the requirements of the medical studies, we were forced to employ the most drastic quota system within the history of the German university. At the University of Freiburg, where I am working, the enrollment of students in medicine has doubled twice in only few years. It is understandable that a larger teaching staff and a restricted enlargement of rooms can not keep pace with such a development. Therefore it was inevitable that lecture halls, course rooms, and patient rooms became more and more crowded. In some cases this was unbearable, especially for the patients. Acceptance of all applicants simply became impossible; therefore the quota became an absolute necessity. This becomes very clear if one keeps in mind that the number of applications for medical studies in Freiburg, for example, is now thirty times greater than the number of places available.

It may seem that I have presented an unpleasant picture of medical care and medical studies in West Germany. But these are the realities with which we are confronted every day. The world needs in great number trained doctors who are well educated both in theory and practice. We have reached a point where necessity and the possibility of its realization have broken. We would need milliards of German Marks to build the educational institutes for those people who would like to study medicine. We would need the same amount of money to build modern hospitals planned for the future and available to all people. We still strive to maintain the traditionally high standard of medicine in Germany, we must accept and recognize this as natural. The system of German medicine still occupies the high rank in world prestige that it achieved through the scientific and medical traditions of the last hundred years. But it has become a hard job to maintain this rank, both for the present and for the future.

SELECTED REFERENCES

Adam, Wilhelm: *Modernes Krankenhaus. Schriftenreihe Fortschrittliche Kommunalverwaltung.* Bd. 18. 3 Aufl. 1973, Köln und Berlin: G. Grote.

Clade, Harald: *Das kranke Krankenhaus. Reform der inneren Struktur.* 1973, Köln: Deutsche Industrieverlags-Gmbh.

Elsholz, Konrad: *Krankenhäuser, Stiefkinder der Wohlstandsgesellschaft.* 1969, Baden-Baden: Nomos Verlagsgesellschaft.

Rohde, Johann Jürgen: *Soziologie des Krankenhauses.* 2 Aufl. 1974, Stuttgart: Enke.

Schäfer, Hans und Blohmke, Maria: *Sozialmedizin.* 1972, Stuttgart: Thieme.

Seidler, Eduard: *Geschichte der Pflege des kranken Menschen.* 3 Aufl. 1972, Stuttgart: Kohlhammer.

The reader will find in the above-mentioned titles broad lists of further publications.

Chapter 6

THE PROVISION OF MEDICAL CARE IN THE COMMUNITY IN THE FEDERAL REPUBLIC OF GERMANY

THOMAS ZICKGRAF
Cologne, Germany

1. The Organization

PRIVATE AND social health insurance offer everybody in Germany a medical service that corresponds to the development in modern medicine as well as to personal needs and intentions. About 90% of the population is covered by the social health insurance.

The social health insurance itself consists of different self-governing bodies ('Krankenkassen'). There are 1645 different 'Krankenkassen' working in certain regions or for certain groups of professions as well as for certain industrial or trade-firms. Doctors in the community working in the social health insurance system—we shall use the term 'panel-doctor' for this group being aware that this term has a different meaning in the NHS in the United Kingdom—are integrated into regional self-governing bodies, the 'Kassenärztliche Vereinigungen'.

Medical care in the community covered by the social health insurance is based on the principles of joint self-government by doctors and social health insurance in the principal organization of the system of medical care by agreement on contracts between social health insurance bodies and Kassenärztliche Vereinigungen, by constituting general directions of a federal joint committee of doctors and Krankenkassen, and by the activities of mutual committees for the admission of doctors to the panel, for control of the economical side of medical treatment, for collective bargaining on remuneration, and arbitration committees. Legal commission of the Kassenärztliche Vereinigungen to secure medical care in the community ('Sicherstellungsauftrag') according to the law of panel-doctors ('Kassenarztrecht') and the principles agreed upon by the self-government. It is also based on the autonomy of contracts between insurance bodies and Kassenärztliche Vereinigungen in an equal partnership between Krankenkassen and panel-doctors in the organization of medical care.

On the federal level only general directions are fixed between Krankenkassen and doctors by the federal joint committee. Since both Krankenkassen and Kassenärztliche Vereinigungen are autonomous bodies they can agree on certain medical measures also by regional agreements.

Doctors are renumerated on a fee for service base. The federal government has set a schedule of fees, with its latest issue in 1965. This schedule is valid for treatments outside social health insurance, unless direct agreements between doctor and patient are made. Doctors may multiply the basic fee up to six times according to the circumstances of the case and the economical state of the patient. The schedule of fees is also valid for the social health insurance but can be varied by contracts between Krankenkasse and Kassenärztlicher Vereinigung. In the moment for instance there are negotiations to cut down the fees for laboratory tests achieved by autoanalysers. Every year there is a regional bargaining on the percentage paid for every single item. This bargaining takes place between the single Krankenkasse and the regional Kassenärztliche Vereinigung. The results vary regionally and also from Krankenkasse to Krankenkasse according to their economical capacity.

This system enables the patient to choose his doctor freely. Admission to special medical services is possible by referring the patient to a specialist through the family doctor or the attending doctor. But the patient may also directly visit a specialist of his choice. Only for hospital treatment patients must be referred by a panel-doctor.

Doctors are obliged to all necessary treatment including diagnostic and therapeutic measures, medical prescriptions, attestation of temporary disablement and reference to hospital care. But they are also obliged to be aware of economic conduct. The economic side of treatment is controlled, as mentioned before, by joint committees.

While the patient in the social health insurance gets medical service entirely free, also the doctor has no financial transactions with the social health insurance bodies. The settlement of accounts is done by his Kassenärztliche Vereinigung.

A few words must be said about the control of economic treatment. The Krankenkassen can apply to the Kassenärztliche Vereinigung for an examination of any panel-doctor's performances, prescriptions, hospital admissions, and disablement-attestations. A committee of doctors then scrutinizes the situation. They can cut down the remuneration or make the doctor pay back a certain sum for uneconomical prescriptions. The judgement of economic conduct is usually done on the average that the same group of doctors spent in that region. But if it comes to discussions, all the other factors, mentioned before, have to be taken into consideration. The afflicted doctor may oppose to such measures and go to court if there is no settlement. The whole business is sometimes quite painful for all the participants, and it is often difficult to find proper measures of what is necessary and economic and what exceeds it. Very often doctors also won't argue, even if they may be right. But the measure in itself is inevitable in the system.

According to the 'Sicherstellungsauftrag' which entitles and obliges the Kassenärztliche Vereinigungen to secure medical care in the community, hospitals have no direct part in this system, they have no out-patient departments. Only university hospitals can treat a restricted number of out-patients for teaching purposes. But according to the exigencies of equal medical care, doctors employed in hospitals may participate personally in the medical care system of the panel-doctors. For special medical services they often get a limited personal admission with the same rights and obligations as the panel-doctors.

Thanks to the partnership between doctors and insurance bodies by joint self-government there has lately never been any conflict to such an extent that could have led to serious disorders in the medical care in the community. This had happened in former times when panel-doctors had immediate contracts to the individual insurance bodies and got into dependence upon them. But it has to be said that doctors have a slightly stronger position against the great number of Krankenkassen.

A great problem, like in most countries, are the tremendously rising expenses for the social health insurance. The social health insurance spent a total of 29.6 milliards DM in 1971 and 34.5 in 1972. The figures for 1973 will be about 40 milliards DM.

Of the total in 1972 30% were spent for hospital care, 24.3% for medical care in the community except dental care, and 18.4% for pharmaceutical products.

While in 1968 hospitals and doctors had the same percentage of 26.6 each, the expenses for hospital care are now growing with an annual augmentation beyond 20%, for pharma products of 14% and for doctors of 10%. The annual average for each person insured amounts to app. DM 600.—in 1972.

2. *Provision of Medical Care*

The Federal Republic of Germany has almost the highest number of doctors according to population of all the European countries. For a population of about 62 million there are 48,200 panel doctors and another 7,400 personally admitted doctors while for medical care in the community there is 1 doctor per 1,115 inhabitants. Also about

50% of the panel-doctors are general practitioners with an average age of 56.1 years. Specialists in established practice have an average age of 51.5 years. Although there is certainly no deficiency of doctors according to absolute numbers, the distribution greatly varies regionally and according to medical discipline.

Until 1960 admittance to the panel by the Kassenärztliche Vereinigung was not free. It depended on a certain ratio formula according to members of the social health insurance in a certain area. This procedure was then declared unconstitutional by the Supreme Court, with the consequence that every established doctor has to be admitted to the panel as long as he fulfills certain requirements in regard to his person. So the Kassenärztliche Vereinigungen now have no direct influence on the establishment of doctors. Quite naturally there is a certain lack of doctors in unattractive regions such as in rural and suburban areas. This situation will not be overcome by an increase in absolute numbers of doctors. Therefore, the Kassenärztliche Vereinigungen have taken serious efforts to encourage the establishment of doctors in these districts in their own liberal practice by financial warrants, loans with low interest, supply of locum tenens, allowance for medical assistants and many others.

The Federal Government is also preparing legal measures by means of which local authorities, social health insurance and Kassenärztliche Vereinigungen will be obliged and enabled to establish proper determination of regional requirements. Only if all measures of the Kassenärztliche Vereinigungen fail to fulfill the requirements, certain restrictions of an entirely free establishment are going to take place.

Since the number of doctors is growing every year, there will soon be an increase in the establishment of doctors throughout the country.

A far greater problem is the unequal distribution between different categories of doctors. The stagnation of the number of general practitioners has led to some trouble in the provision of primary medical care in regions where there are not enough specialists to cover these needs.

The German Medical Association has established a postgraduate education programme for general practitioners. But a lot more has to be done to establish family medicine in the university-teaching-programmes to motivate students to this important branch of medical activities.

Insufficient is especially the psychiatric care. The absolute number of specialists in this field is not sufficient. By special agreements between Kassenärztliche Vereinigungen and social health insurance it was possible to let psychoanalytically based non-medical psychotherapists participate in the treatment under the social health insurance scheme.

3. Quality of Medical Care

The legal commission of the Kassenärztliche Vereinigungen to secure medical care in the community entitles only established doctors to take part in the treatment under social health insurance. This has led to a fully developed system of both general practice and special medical services in established practices outside the hospitals. It gives patients the opportunity of free access to the doctors of their confidence.

The fee for service remuneration system enables doctors to keep up an adequate technical equipment for both diagnostic and therapeutic measures. This is naturally more so with specialists, but also the general practitioner has in many cases an ECG, a certain laboratory outfit, and sometimes X-ray equipment.

To secure a standard of quality for the technical performances the Kassenärztliche Vereinigungen have set conditions to be fulfilled for X-ray equipment as well as for personal X-ray training. For laboratory tests a quality-control system has just been established.

The growing necessity of technical equipment also leads doctors to new forms of cooperation. In the Federal Republic the individual practicing doctor is still the rule. But more and more doctors tend to use expensive medical equipment in groups and different forms of cooperations.

A certain disadvantage of this system is the rather strict separation between medical practice in hospitals and in the community. This can and often does cause a lack of communication with the result of sometimes unnecessary repetition of diagnostic measures. After discharge from the hospital there might be a gap in continuity of medical care and also, if panel-doctors do not cooperate properly, there is unnecessary admission to hospitals for diagnostic and therapeutic procedures that might just as well be carried out by established doctors at much lower expense.

The growing expense for medical care in the social health insurance has led to heavy criticism against the 'Sicherstellungsauftrag' of the Kassenärztliche Vereinigungen. It is estimated a mere monopoly for panel-doctors with a terrific waste of medical resources among political parties and trade unions.

The solution is seen in opening hospitals for medical care in the community outside the panel-doctors system. A more radical proposal by the trade unions promotes so-called integrated medical systems in which all the technical performances should be centralized in technical centres, equally used by hospitals and panel-doctors, in order to minimize expenses for maximum of efficiency at a high standard of quality. Furthermore this system is supposed to unburden doctors from merely technical performances in order to give them more time for their patients.

The idea behind these propositions is also the belief of improving preventive medicine by more or less unselected screening methods which would be carried out large scale through an automated laboratory equipment.

In our opinion the medical result of a development of that sort is more than doubtful, not to speak of the economical outcome. The necessary concentration of these technical centers and as an immediate consequence also of specialists in towns with a certain amount of population would also include many inconveniences for patients of less populated areas.

The solution sought by the Kassenärztliche Vereinigungen is to encourage rationalization in medical practice and cooperation between panel-doctors in different forms of group-practicing on the understanding that the personal relationship between the patient and his doctor should not be impaired.

There are also plans of keeping an eye on hospital-admissions by panel-doctors in order to use to full extent the possibilities of established doctors before a patient is admitted for hospital care. For further improvement of cooperation between hospital doctors and panel-doctors, specialists in hospitals are personally admitted to medical care in the community under social health insurance where it is required for the medical care of the population. This we consider more effectful for the patient then to establish out-patient departments in the hospitals.

On the other side panel-doctors should be enabled to treat their own patients in hospitals. But there is a strong tendency against that in the organizations of social health insurance bodies and hospitals.

With the enormous increase in demand for medical services the established doctors are very often overburdened. According to a recent interrogation of patients most complaints about medical care in the community were put forward against the long times one had to spend in doctors' waiting rooms. Dentists have solved this problem successfully by a strict appointment-system. In general practice this is much more difficult.

4. Preventive Medicine

Three years ago certain programmes for the prevention of some illnesses have been introduced into the social health insurance scheme. They are yet limited to diagnostic programmes for cancer of the female breast, cancer of rectum and prostata and collum carcinoma. Besides there are maternity- and early childhood-programmes.

The programmes are based on the following principles: The illness must be effectively treatable; early states of the illness must be recognizable by diagnostic measures; the symptoms must be clearly identified by medical technical means, there must be a sufficient number of doctors and institutions to perform adequate diagnosis and treatment of all suspicious cases.

The establishment of preventive measures means an important change in the task and items of social health insurance from merely curative medicine to a health control system. Unfortunately the response of our population is so far very poor. Only the check-ups during pregnancy and the early childhood programme were called upon to some substantial extent with great variation though according to social status. With respect to the rather high childbirth mortality in the Federal Republic there has not been a remarkable success in this field. The cancer programmes are used only by about 25 to 50% of the females and 10 to 20% of the males, again with a wide range according to social status.

5. Emergency Services

Panel-doctors are supposed to be present for their patients during the night and they are obliged to participate in an emergency service of their home town or villages on weekends. Dispensation from this obligation is possible for personal reasons. Specialists must participate in the service and very rarely get dispensation on behalf of their specialization. In some country areas the doctors on duty for weekends have radio equipment in their cars in order to save time and to be always ready for urgent calls.

This kind of service covers more than 90% of the emergency cases, only about 3% go to hospital for treatment. In some cities it was necessary to establish an organized emergency service with a central emergency call station, where a doctor is present. Taxi-cabs take doctors to the patients and summon calls from the central station. In this service hospital-doctors participate voluntarily. They are also paid fee for service.

The German States are just now passing so called rescue-legislation in order to organize an emergency service throughout the country for taking care of traffic and other accidents and seriously ill patients. The organization will be in the hands of the Red Cross and other charitable organizations.

Conclusion

Summing up we can say that to our opinion the organization of medical care in the community based on the principles of self-government between the social health insurance bodies and the doctors' organizations, the Kassenärztliche Vereinigungen, based on autonomy of contracts and on the legal commission of the Kassenärztliche Vereinigungen to secure medical care in the community, was able to meet the exigencies of the population according to their personal needs and with regard to the development of modern medicine. The system is flexible enough to fulfill all these needs in the future and to perform the necessary reforms through contracts and agreements between the insurance bodies and the doctors' organizations.

Chapter 7

MANPOWER PROBLEMS IN THE MEDICAL CARE SYSTEM IN CANADA

J. R. EVANS
Toronto University, Toronto, Canada

UNDER CANADA's federal system, primary responsibility for health and education reside at provincial level. The size, needs and resources of the ten provinces vary considerably and this has been reflected in differences of approach to the organization of health services and in the timing of introduction of programmes such as health insurance. In spite of these differences, however, the outcome has been surprisingly consistent throughout Canada and potential disparities between provinces have been minimized by federal guidelines linked with financial incentives to the provinces.

The national health plan in Canada evolved in stages over two decades. In 1948 the National Health Grant programme made available funds for hospital construction in anticipation of public hospital insurance which was introduced on a national basis in 1958. Following on the Report of the Royal Commission on Health Services, the federal Health Resources Fund was established in 1965 to expand the supply of health manpower in anticipation of medicare. And, in 1968 the federal programme of publicly sponsored and administered medical care insurance came into effect. All necessary medical services are now covered by health insurance except dental services and prescription drugs. The health insurance is portable, universal, prepaid and there are no limits on the medical benefits covered. The plans are financed primarily from tax revenue, although in some provinces there are premiums for those with taxable income above a certain level.

The introduction of national health insurance has not been associated with any outward change in the ownership of hospitals or in the private practice of medicine. There is no distinction between private and public hospital beds other than the non-medical amenities for which supplementary private insurance can be obtained. Similarly there is no distinction between private medical practice and practice under the publicly sponsored insurance plan. Most practising physicians are paid for both hospital and office work on a fee for service basis in accordance with a fee schedule negotiated in each province between the government and the provincial medical association.

One sector of health policy which has received much less emphasis in Canada is health research. The growth of biomedical research and technology has been much slower than in the United States and its impact on education of the health professions and on teaching hospitals has been much less extensive. During the past five years special funds have been made available by government for research on problems associated with the cost, quality and distribution of health services and the evaluation of innovations in the delivery of health care.

With universal health insurance and with a well developed, perhaps over developed, system of hospital services the principal problems in the delivery of health care to the community are the organization of health services and the distribution of health manpower. For government the overriding problem is control of costs. International comparisons indicate that Canada, like Sweden and the United States spends over seven percent of gross national product on health services. Hospital expenditures account for nearly two-thirds of health costs and, since hospitals are financed directly by provincial government agencies, restraints have been imposed in the form of ceilings on expenditure and reduction in the number of beds. With these measures the overall rate of increase in health costs has been held to about twelve percent per annum, but the wage settlements in 1974 will have a profound inflationary effect. This will lead to renewed pressure for economies in other parts of the system and for the development of alternatives to the use of expensive inpatient facilities of active treatment hospitals.

Although hospital costs are the largest single category of public expenditure on health, one of the most important determinants of total health costs is the number and type of physicians practising in the system. Since the physician decides admission to hospital, duration of stay, use of diagnostic and therapeutic procedures, referrals and the pattern of further examination it has been estimated that costs attributable to physicians represents nearly eighty percent of total health costs. It follows that a surplus of doctors, particularly procedurally orientated specialists, will increase the cost of health services without necessarily improving health. The increase in costs results in part from the additional fees for service but to a much greater extent from the steering effect of their pattern of practice on diagnostic services and hospital expenditures. This matter is of immediate concern in provinces where a surplus of physicians is imminent or already exists.

The overwhelming preoccupation of government and the health

profession with the delivery of health services has obscured the more fundamental issue of preservation of health and attack on the more fundamental root causes of disease. With the advance of biomedical science it has become increasingly clear that much illness is self inflicted by patterns of individual and group behaviour. The attack on problems of life style—diet, exercise, personal habits— and on problems of the environment for living—housing, crowding, anonymity, pollution—involves education of the public to adopt new patterns of behaviour. The white paper entitled 'A New Perspective on the Health of Canadians' recently published in Canada by the Minister of National Health (Lalonde, 1974) analyzes the problem and outlines a possible strategy for attack. Development of the instruments for implementation of this strategy should be given the highest priority since success in this area has the greatest promise of improving health and at the same time reducing the rate of escalation of expenditures on health services.

Organization of Health Services

Almost all regions in Canada are adequately supplied with active treatment hospital beds; the ratio is over five beds per 1,000 population in all provinces and considerably higher in some. In contrast, until very recently there have been inadequate beds for chronically ill and convalescent patients and for the care of the elderly in most provinces and no proper alternatives to hospitalization for many patients who could have been managed on an outpatient basis. Furthermore, there has been no mechanism for coordinating the planning of services among hospitals in the same community or region. The strong identification of lay boards of trustees and medical staff with their own hospitals, and the desire to have each institution totally self-sufficient, have impeded cooperative planning among hospitals and resulted in a certain amount of wasteful competition and duplication of specialized facilities.

Two courses of action have now been taken. The authorized level for active treatment hospital beds has been reduced in some provinces by about twenty percent and, at the same time, financial assistance has been offered to make available more accommodation for chronic and convalescent care. Secondly, a comprehensive approach to the planning and management of health services on an area-wide basis has been adopted by all the provinces. Regional or district health councils have been established as an intermediate structure between the individual hospital or institution and the provincial government department or hospital commission. To date these bodies have been advisory only but in most areas they have made considerable progress on a voluntary basis towards the rationalization of hospital services and the achievement of better balance for the full spectrum of health services in the region. In other areas, for example the large metropolitan centres, voluntary cooperation has been more difficult to achieve and the major problems are unlikely to be resolved until more formal structures for regional administration are established with authority to set priorities and allocate resources according to community needs.

From the standpoint of the individual citizen the most obvious need for improved organization relates to primary or first line health care for ambulatory patients in the communities in which they live. In Canada primary health services are delivered by physicians most of whom are in solo office practice or small groups. In areas where there is a shortage of physicians, or where physicians do not provide services at night or on weekends, there is increasing dependence on hospital emergency rooms for primary care. A recent survey in Ontario (Pickering, 1973) noted that public complaints about accessibility and availability of primary care, fragmentation of services, lack of continuity of care and the impersonal manner in which services are delivered are not widespread but are sufficiently common that they cannot be disregarded. Since primary care represents about eighty percent of all health services, it is not surprising that these characteristics strongly influence the public perception of quality of care and lead to the conclusion of deteriorating quality at a time when by professional and scientific standards quality of care has never been higher. The missing element of structure in primary care is an organizational framework to coordinate the contributions of the different health professionals and agencies in a community and as a mechanism for shifting the balance from disease-oriented, hospital-based care to health maintenance and the management of disability outside the institutional setting.

The advantages of better organization of primary care services are widely recognized but there has been reluctance to proceed with formal community health centres on a broad scale. Provincial governments fear additional cost, doctors are apprehensive about organizational constraints on professional freedom and conflict with consumer dominated management groups, and for citizens with complete financial coverage under national health insurance there is little incentive to promote community health centres except where a shortage of doctors exists. A federal government proposal in 1973 to finance community health centres with a special 'thrust fund' was sidetracked in debate over federal-provincial financial transfers. A number of centres have been established by medical schools for teaching purposes but widespread application of the concept is unlikely to occur until there is special financial support from government and a designated sponsor or organizational focus in the community.

To recapitulate, the resources for community health have evolved in a highly individualistic way. The system of health services consists of a large number of isolated health professionals and separately supported hospitals and agencies operating more or less independently. But rising costs and rising public expectations in a publicly financed health system have forced attention on the need to coordinate these resources to provide a more balanced and comprehensive range of services to the community on a more efficient economical basis. This process of change involves new organizational arrangements and a much greater sharing of responsibility by doctors with other doctors, with other health professionals and with the public who receive and finance the services.

Recruitment and Migration of Physicians

Responding to the report of the Royal Commission on Health Services, the federal government established in 1965 a Health Resources Fund of twenty-five dollars per capita to be spent over fifteen years to assist the provinces with the expansion and up-grading of facilities for education of the health professions and for medical research. Since 1965 four new medical schools have come into operation and most of the existing twelve medical schools have been expanded to achieve more than a doubling of capacity for undergraduate and postgraduate medical education. When the benefit of this expansion is fully realized in 1978, the medical schools will graduate 1742 doctors per year, and Canada should be self-sufficient with respect to medical manpower.

Since 1965 the supply of physicians has increased much more rapidly than was anticipated and the physician : population ratio is now close to 1 : 600. The unexpectedly rapid increase has been due to the immigration of foreign medical graduates which for the period from 1965 to 1970 exceeded the output of our own medical schools. If immigration of physicians continues at the current rate of 1,000 per year and there is no change in enrolment patterns in Canadian medical schools, the number of physicians in Canada will continue to increase at a much greater rate than population and the ratio projected for 1981 will be 1 : 488.

Of the physicians active in practice in 1972, thirty-one percent were graduates of foreign medical schools. Table I shows that the proportion of foreign medical graduates in general practice (32 percent) was slightly greater than in the aggregate of all specialties

(28 percent). But among the specialties, Psychiatry, Anaesthesia and several of the small specialties had a higher than average percentage of foreign medical graduates. The relatively large number of foreign medical graduates in internship and residency posts (37 percent) may be explained by the licensing requirement of two years' experience in an approved Canadian training programme. (This requirement is waived for graduates of accredited medical schools in the United States and those fully registered with the General Medical Council of Great Britain.)

Table I

Active Canadian and Foreign Medical Graduates by Specialty, 1972

	Canadian	Foreign	Total
General Practice	9,028	4,305	13,333
Total Specialists	11,044	4,233	15,277
Internal Medicine	1,743	487	2,230
General Surgery	1,615	457	2,072
Surgical Specialties*	1,004	286	1,290
Psychiatry	910	466	1,376
Anaesthesia	837	372	1,209
Obstetrics and Gynaecology	843	279	1,122
Radiology	752	315	1,067
Other	3,340	1,571	4,911
Interns and Residents	3,709	2,189	5,898
TOTAL	23,781	10,727	34,508

* Excluding Ophthalmologists and Otolaryngologists.

Source: Health Manpower Planning Division, Health and Welfare Directory 1973. Based on data extracted from Canadian Medical Directory Tape, January, 1973.

The origin of the foreign medical graduates is also of interest. Figure I indicates the last country of residence of physicians immigrating to Canada each year from 1961 to 1972. Countries accounting for five percent or more of the foreign medical graduates registered in that year are identified and the remainder are pooled in the category 'other countries'. Significant immigration occurred from India, 'China' (chiefly Hong Kong), Turkey, the Philippines, the Irish Republic and the West Indies for several years in each case during the period. The only two countries of origin which were consistently represented each year were Great Britain and the United States. The relatively high figures for Great Britain, ranging from 25 to 35 percent, however, may be misleading in recent years since a considerable number of the immigrants were graduates of Asian medical schools who trained or practised in Great Britain before emigrating to Canada.

IMMIGRANT PHYSICIANS BY COUNTRY OF FORMER RESIDENCE IN PERCENTAGE FORM.

MÉDECINS IMMIGRANTS PAR PAYS DE DERNIÈRE RÉSIDENCE, PRÉSENTÉ EN POURCENTAGE

1961 - 1972

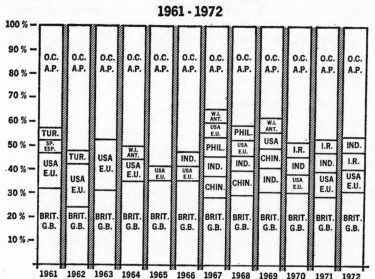

O.C. - OTHER COUNTRIES
A.P. - AUTRES PAYS

Fig. 1. Former country of residence of foreign medical graduates immigrating to Canada between 1961 and 1972. (*Source:* Health Manpower Planning Division, Health and Welfare Canada, 1973.)

Key: BRIT. = Great Britain
CHIN. = China (Hong Kong, Taiwan and Mainland China)
IND. = India
I.R. = Irish Republic
PHIL. = Philippines
SP. = Spain
TUR. = Turkey
USA = United States of America
W.I. = West Indies
O.C. = Other countries contributing less that five percent to total immigration in that year.

Returning to the problem of geographic distribution of physicians, the overall figures for supply mask major differences between regions. Figure II compares the ratio of physicians to population in each of the ten provinces and in Canada as a whole. Prince Edward Island, Newfoundland and New Brunswick still lag well behind the national average and have only about half as many physicians per capita as one of the more affluent provinces, British Columbia. Furthermore, manpower studies in the favoured provinces show major interregional differences and many communities have been

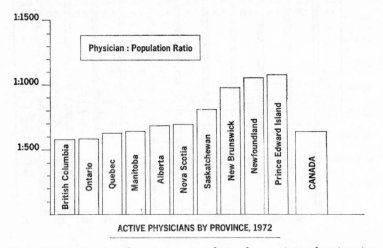

ACTIVE PHYSICIANS BY PROVINCE, 1972

Fig. 2. Ratio of active physicians to population by province of registration in 1972 (*Source:* Health Manpower Planning Division, Health and Welfare Canada, 1973.)

identified which are underserviced, particularly in the sparsely populated areas. At the same time other communities are now faced with actual or impending oversupply.

The principal response to shortages in Canada has been the effort to increase the overall supply of physicians and other health personnel through expanded educational programmes. New medical schools established in Newfoundland and Quebec resulted in improvements in the local region even before graduates emerged. Some medical schools have started more specific programmes to provide clinical experience for residents and senior undergraduates in underserviced regions with the hope of attracting these individuals back to practise in such regions. In some regions incentives have been offered to attract physicians to practise in underserviced areas. In Ontario there has been an excellent response to a programme including return-of-service bursaries for medical students, establishment of practice grants for suitable facilities and guaranteed minimum income at an attractive level during the initial years of practice. In the Yukon Territory the shortage of doctors has been partially overcome by offering remuneration at 120 percent of the fee schedule in British Columbia. Most of these incentive programmes, however, only deal with the primary level of care in grossly underserviced areas. The overall pattern of distribution of manpower remains very uneven and there are many regions which lack the services of medical specialists.

The problems of manpower distribution are further complicated by the proliferation of health professions and by the differentiation of individual professions into generalists and specialists of different types. Both processes tend to divide medical care into a series of compartments or territories, each identified with a single profession or specialty, rather than with the overall objectives of health care. Fortunately, there has been no attempt in Canada to introduce new categories of health personnel comparable to the physician's assistant in the United States. Rather than introduce a new professional entity, experienced nurses have been given the equivalent of six months' additional training to prepare them to work with physicians in the delivery of primary care in the office setting.

The process of specialization in medicine, however, is well established in Canada. In the past decade the number of specialists has increased by 70 percent while the number of general practitioners has increased by only 19 percent but data obtained in December, 1972 indicates that nearly half the doctors in active practice were still in general practice (Table I). During the past five years there has been a change in student interests and an increasing proportion of Canadian medical graduates have entered general practice or family medicine. Departments of family or community medicine have been established in all our medical schools, postgraduate training opportunities for primary care physicians have been greatly expanded and rationing of the number of specialty training posts has commenced in some provinces. These educational efforts to reverse the earlier trend towards specialization have been supported at the national level by the vigorous educational programme of the Canadian College of Family Practice and by the policy of restraint on proliferation of new specialties exercised by the Royal College of Physicians and Surgeons of Canada.

An important question is the extent to which the prospect of a higher level of renumeration influenced medical graduates in their selection of general or specialty practice as a career. Table II compares the average net professional income of general practitioners

Table II

INDICES—AVERAGE NET PROFESSIONAL INCOME

	1966	1971	New Placing
General Practice	100	100	
Orthopaedics	185.2	158.1	(1)
Neurosurgery	183.8	148.1	(4)
Otology	171.9	152.7	(3)
Radiology	166.6	141.1	(9)
Plastic Surgery	156.7	155.2	(2)
Urology	155.5	141.6	(7)
Ophthal.	155.5	141.4	(8)
Thoracic Surgery	150.4	144.5	(6)
General Surgery	138.5	127.5	(12)
Derm.	135.7	133.4	(10)
Obs. and Gyn.	133.5	146.0	(5)
Pathology	129.6	131.2	(11)
Anaesth.	119.9	111.9	(13)
Int. Med.	113.0	106.4	(15)
Psych.	108.1	95.4	(16)
Paed.	107.6	106.9	(14)
All Specialists	134.5	126.7	

with different types of specialists. In 1966, general practitioners received the lowest income of all groups which was only about 60 percent of the average income of the top surgical specialties. By 1971 the relative position of the general practitioner had improved chiefly because of the considerable narrowing of the range of incomes but still the general practitioner was at the lower end of the scale together with the psychiatrist, internist and paediatrician. With a fee-for-service system and historically based fee schedules the surgeons and medical specialists who carry out technical procedures are favoured financially. The justification for significant differences in income between the various branches of medicine is doubtful but if there is to be a differential, the current perspective of needs suggests that it should favour practitioners whose skills are with people rather than with techniques. The prospect of higher remuneration undoubtedly influences some medical graduates in their choice of specialty but this alone fails to explain the lack of interest in general practice during the 1960's because during that period internal medicine and paediatrics with comparable levels of remuneration were popular career choices. It seems likely that intellectual stimulation, interest in people, environment of practice and other factors were also important considerations.

Medical schools have an important role in the process of

rationalizing the supply of primary care physicians and specialists of different types. By agreement with the Royal College of Physicians and Surgeons of Canada which controls all specialty examinations, full responsibility for the planning, organization and supervision of all residency training leading to specialty qualifications was transferred in 1965 from individual hospitals to university medical centres. In some provinces guidelines have been established for the number of postgraduate trainees eligible for provincial support and priorities have been recommended for certain types of trainees. In Ontario, for example, the number of residency training posts associated with each medical school is limited to a number equivalent to its undergraduate enrolment. Opportunities for postgraduate training in primary care must be provided for at least fifty percent of medical graduates and the remaining places are for the various specialties. Quebec has recently adopted a similar scheme and furthermore has placed a quota of fifteen percent on foreign medical graduates in postgraduate training programs to become effective in 1976.

The medical manpower strategy followed in Canada to date relies almost exclusively on changes in the output of undergraduate and postgraduate educational programs. This approach is unlikely to be successful for a number of reasons. Firstly, major changes in educational programs such as the establishment of a new school or training program involve a long lead time. The interval between recognition of the need and the appearance of graduates in significant numbers from the program is rarely less than seven years and often longer. Secondly, manpower forecasting is notoriously unreliable and involves many variables which are not controlled by the educational system, e.g. changes in the incidence or management of disease, the role of other health professions, the methods of delivering health care, or the rewards from different types of practice. Thirdly, uneven geographic distribution of health personnel can only be influenced to a very limited extent by changes in the educational programs. The evidence to date suggests that increases in the supply of physicians alone is not sufficient to overcome the major interregional differences in medical manpower. Finally, solutions to the manpower problems which are devised in our medical schools will almost certainly prove to be ineffective when half of the new physicians registered each year in Canada have been trained in other countries. If our manpower policies are to be based primarily on the regulation of supply, then these policies must relate to both sources of supply, our medical schools and immigration.

If we are to resolve the serious inequities of distribution of physicians by type and geographic location, the emphasis must

shift from a supply strategy to policies which influence the utilization or deployment of health personnel. The principal mechanism
used to date to overcome shortages has been the 'supersaturation-
spillover approach' which is extremely costly and relatively ineffective. Special incentives have been used with some success in
certain provinces as a short term measure to attract general practitioners to underserviced areas, but incentives are most useful for
shortages and in the long run a method is required which will deal
not only with shortages but also with the problem of oversupply.
In British Columbia and Ontario the physician : population ratio
is already well under 1 : 600 and may be expected to reach 1 : 500
within the next few years if the current sources of supply continue
unabated.

The surplus of medical manpower may at first glance seem
attractive, particularly to economists, but more careful examination
reveals several undesirable consequences. First, it will lead to substantial and unnecessary increase in health costs since the number of
doctors in practice is probably the most important determinant of
total expenditures on health services. This is particularly true if the
surplus consists of a large number of hospital-based specialists.
Secondly, the effective workload per doctor will be reduced and this,
in turn, may decrease the quality of services rendered and reduce
the level of professional satisfaction. The effect of an inadequate case
load in open heart surgical units on the mortality rate and cost
of surgery is well known. A similar problem may exist in other
specialties. For example, the ratio of neurosurgeons to population
is four times as great in British Columbia as it is in Newfoundland,
but the number of major neurosurgical procedures per capita is
approximately the same in the two provinces. Thirdly, in addition
to decreasing productivity, a surplus of doctors may displace other
professions from their role in the delivery of health services.

Due to the recent expansion, Canadian medical schools can now
train sufficient physicians to maintain, and even improve, our
physician : population ratio without dependence on immigration. If
a future surplus of physicians is to be avoided, it now seems
necessary to make a choice either to limit immigration or to reduce
the output of our medical schools. With established capacity in our
medical schools, with a surplus of well qualified Canadian applicants
(1,178 acceptable Canadian applicants were turned away in 1972
and a higher number in 1973) and with specific manpower objectives
concerning the balance between generalists and specialists and
representation of women, native peoples and ethnic groups, there
are abundant reasons for not reducing the output of our medical
schools. But as long as shortages exist in some regions of Canada and

in specific branches of medicine there will be strong public resistance and valid professional objections to placing rigid restrictions on immigration.

An alternative approach which copes with the problem of over-supply of physicians and at the same time favourably influences redistribution to underserviced areas is the establishment of 'upper limits' on the number of physicians by geographic region and by the type of general or specialty practice in which they engage. The upper limits should be in accord with guidelines developed by provincial or national manpower advisory councils and should be subject to regular review and modification. Physicians would be required to apply for practice privileges to a regional or district health council in the same way as individual physicians now apply for hospital privileges. The manpower limits might be applied for the province as a whole through the existing licensing machinery but this would be less effective in meeting the need for equitable distribution of physicians among the various regions of the province. Individual regions should retain some authority to substitute between different types of physicians and other health personnel or to exceed the established limits by cutting back on other health expenditures if this seemed more appropriate to local needs. Implementation of the concept would require the establishment of regional authorities with much greater knowledge of and responsibility for health services of that area and more sophisticated information on the appropriate numbers of physicians of different types and the nature of the practice in which they engage.

Although restraints are much less acceptable in Canada than incentives as a method of influencing human behaviour, the concept of upper limits on the establishment of physicians in a particular area has enough advantages to warrant careful consideration. Firstly, it is an important measure in achieving optimal geographic distribution of general practitioners and specialists in relation to regional needs. Secondly, it is a major factor in solving the problem of cost control since a surplus of physicians, particularly hospital based specialists, leads to increased expenditures without significant improvement in health. Thirdly, it links changes in medical manpower to the evolution of patterns of practice and to the involvement of other types of health personnel. Fourthly, it provides a firmer basis for manpower forecasts as a guide to those responsible for planning the programs of basic and specialized professional education. And finally, with such a system Canadian or foreign medical graduates can be considered for vacancies in a region on the basis of their professional qualifications thereby obviating the need to introduce rigid restrictions on immigration.

At the federal-provincial conference of Health Ministers in February, 1974 consensus was reached on a collaborative policy to achieve the following objectives: Firstly, a better balance between the requirements for physicians of all kinds, taking into account the role of allied health workers and the two sources of supply of physicians—Canadian medical schools and immigration. Secondly, to give a higher priority to Canadian students aspiring to a medical career and to Canadian graduates wishing to practise in Canada. Thirdly, to promote a better distribution of physician's services, particularly in rural areas, as well as to relate specialty training to community needs. The Health Ministers indicated that well coordinated measures must soon be taken to achieve these objectives considering the varying circumstances in each province. Some of the options to be considered include physician quota systems by region, appropriate medical school enrolment and restrictions on immigration. The process of consultation with the provinces on preferred mechanisms is already under way and immigration regulations to Canada have been modified to include consideration of occupational demand. If there is no effective demand, the immigrant may not be admitted, but if he has a specific position to fill or is applying to an area with identified vacancies he can be admitted. These new immigration regulations have a general application and are not confined to physicians. The changes which have been introduced make provision for regional underserviced areas and provincial agreement is required before the demand category can be set at zero for Canada.

Emphasis on utilization does not mean that modifications of sources of supply are unimportant. Indeed, they are critical to the type, quality and attitude of future health personnel. For the reasons given, however, manipulation of production machinery alone will not solve the problems unless associated with complementary changes in the utilization machinery. Since the latter has a more immediate effect, it is also a more sensitive method of making ongoing adjustments in response to changing needs.

The author is indebted to Dr. William Hacon, Health Manpower Planning Division, Health and Welfare Canada for much of the data included in this paper.

References

A New Perspective on the Health of Canadians, a working document, Lalonde, Marc, Ottawa, 1974, Government of Canada.
Special Study Regarding the Medical Profession in Ontario, Pickering, Edward A., Toronto, 1973, Ontario Medical Association.

Chapter 8

IMPACT OF HEALTH CARE LEGISLATION ON THE
MEDICAL SCHOOL

M. McGREGOR
McGill University, Montreal, Canada

IN CANADA both health and education are the responsibility of the
ten provinces. However, the initiative for both hospitalization and
medicare came from our federal government. In both instances
Ottawa achieved this by specifying the terms under which it would
participate in payment for such schemes. As a result there are only
minor differences between the present hospital and medicare schemes
in our different provinces and they are available to all Canadians
irrespective of province of residence.

One might anticipate that the removal of financial restraints on
usage would put major strains on the hospitals, on the Medical
Profession and on the Medical Schools. I will indicate that the
strains which might have been expected as a consequence of excess
use of hospitals or of physician's services, have in the event been
relatively small. There have, however, been other and unexpected
consequences of these measures which we must consider.

First let me remind you that the University Medical School has
traditionally been expected to fulfil two quite different roles, roles
which are often in conflict. One, is what I might call the true
University role. This sees the University Medical School as a place
whose business is knowledge, the truth, a place where the truth
is sought after in study, discussion and research; where the truth
is classified and stored and made available. This is a place where both
teacher and student have great freedom to choose their fields of
research and study. Success in this role is measured by research
productivity, by originality, by the evidence of rigorous scientific
criticism and evaluation.

This role has little to do with technical training nor with the
needs of society for technically trained manpower. Thus it is not
measured by the number or technical competence of the doctors
it produces.

Then there is another role, the training role. This is determined by
the need to produce manpower with appropriate technical skills
and in appropriate numbers to fulfil society's needs. Success in this
role is indeed measured by the number and skill and *appropriateness*

of the training of the doctors who emerge from the school. I would suggest that government's involvement in health finances is forcing our schools towards first one role and then the other, and this is, at the least, confusing.

Now they have always had to chose their priorities and in the past they have had considerable freedom of choice. In a free economic system the students were the 'customers' and input was limited by their ability to pay the fees, schools could lean to the University role or to the training role much as they wished. In this way they could differentiate, choose a role and strive for excellence.

Following the Flexner report in 1911 there was a general swing towards the University role but it was still possible for a practitioner orientated school to concentrate most of its effort on training for practice and general practice at that, while at the other extreme a school like Harvard could stress the academic aspects of its role and excel in research.

Not only the universities but also the hospitals, the essential training grounds of our Medical Schools, could choose their direction. All by definition were committed to clinical service. But some could make this virtually their sole role while others elected to commit themselves as well to both medical education and to research.

Thus whatever one's criticism of the laissez faire free enterprise system it certainly provided for a large degree of differentiation and experimentation in the Medical Schools of the western world. But in the last quarter century the scene has changed and the Medical Schools and their hospitals have found themselves beffeted by powerful economic and social forces which have forced them first to accentuate one role and then the other. More important, as the interventions of the state have become greater and more powerful the ability of the Medical Schools to differentiate and experiment has become less.

I presume it is the object of this international symposium to compare notes, to analyze these forces and to decide whether our Medical Schools should change more radically or whether they have already changed too much.

What are these forces? The most obvious is a consequence of the increasing role of the state in both health and education. Twenty-five years ago no more than 2% of the operating funds of my University, McGill, came from the public purse. My hospital, The Royal Victoria Hospital, was also financed principally by patients' fees or by charity. Today, in contrast, 80% of my university's budget comes from direct government grant and my hospital's budget comes almost entirely from the state.

All this has come about relatively peaceably. The outward forms have not been changed. Each institution still has its Board of Governors and its President or its Principal. The 'customers' are still the students or the patients. But the real power, the financial power, has shifted to the state and the state is far more articulate than the students or the patient used to be in expressing its feelings about what Medical Schools and Health Services ought to be. And I must add, just as fickle. And because it wields such power, its changing objectives have far more effect on Medical Education.

I suppose the first major exercise of this power came in the years following World War II. The prevailing social sentiment which caused it was admiration for the achievements of science. This was the 'isn't science wonderful!' epoch. This was most marked in North America and especially in the USA where the demos has always tended to couple its prevailing sentiments with positive action.

Here the money awarded by Congress for research was apparently boundless. And, consistent with its individualistic private enterprise sympathies, its support was awarded to individuals rather than to the institutions in which they worked. Medical School policy, if such there existed in this period, was to give honor to biological research, to attract more successful research workers from each other and to allocate more space to this form of activity. In this way some Medical Schools entered the present decade with over 80% of their operating funds deriving from grants for biological research awarded on a short term basis to successful research workers.

This trend was less marked in Canada and was coupled with a substantial increase in direct government support of university education. Accordingly the balance was better preserved. But the research carrot south of the border was juicy and it was necessary to compete, if only to retain some of our intelligent and ambitious Canadians at home. Thus in 1970, even in Canada, the percent of budget derived from research granting agencies ranged from 10 to as high as 60%.

Now I do not wish to discuss here whether this expenditure on research was too much or too little. My point is that society at this time held biological research in high esteem and that over a 20 year period society used the immense financial power it had concentrated in government to profoundly influence the nature of the North American Medical School. This power was used to force Medical Schools to accentuate the University-Research role often to the detriment of the training role; and it diminished their ability to establish their own policies.

There was a second identifiable social sentiment which began to emerge in the first half of this century. This is the increasingly widespread conviction of society that 'health is a fundamental human right'. This is causing a massive re-accentuation of the training role. The reason, is that this conviction has been coupled with the belief, which I believe to be largely erroneous, that health is to be achieved by free access to what have been miscalled 'health services'.

When the principle scourges of mankind were related to preventable diseases this notion might have had more truth. However, in Europe and North America today I believe health in the true sense of the word has more to do with entirely different factors, factors such as employment, environment, intellectual development and a sense of meaningful involvement in society. The availability of hospitals and doctors and nurses is only a marginal factor in achieving real health in this sense of the word.

Be that as it may, society has decided in most of our countries that provision of these facilities to all citizens is a fundamental right. And to provide this it has been necessary to finance through the state or even to nationalize health services and the health professions and this has been done in the context of otherwise capitalist free enterprise societies. To varying degrees we have removed restraints which previously operated.

With relatively free education we have largely removed economic restraints on those who might wish to enter the medical profession and we have at the same time virtually guaranteed their future incomes at a high level thereafter.

With the state's undertaking to supply health services it becomes more necessary that we should provide enough health professionals with appropriate training. The schools are no longer free to simply offer a variety of training opportunities and leave it to the students to choose what they will do. It is expected that the medical schools will now *produce* the right sort of graduates to fulfil its needs. The very concept of 'producing' a product is contrary to the whole meaning of the University role.

And then by the very nature of the formulae we have chosen to remunerate our doctors we have introduced powerful economic incentives which are influencing the nature of medical practice itself and hence of training. All these changes are affecting our medical schools and their teaching hospitals. Let us consider each of them very briefly.

Free access to our hospitals was provided in Quebec in 1961. As gloomily predicted by many, this was followed by a sharp increase in hospital costs. I am indebted to Professor Lee Soderstrom of the McGill Department of Economics for the figures reflected in Fig. 1. You see that in the five years following free hospitalization hospital operating costs rose by 17.2% per year although the

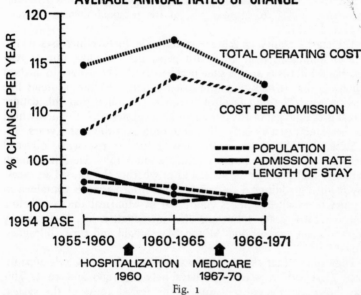

INFLATION IN PUBLIC GENERAL & ALLIED SPECIAL HOSPITALS IN QUEBEC. 1955-1971 (SODERSTROM L.) AVERAGE ANNUAL RATES OF CHANGE

Fig. 1

population in this period was increasing at only 2% per year.

Can one attribute this increase in operating costs to excessive usage? The answer is clearly 'no'. Admission rates rose by 1.3% per year and length of stay per admission rose by 0.5% per year. It would seem that the increased expenditure was the result of an increase in the cost per admission which rose by 13.5% per annum. And this in turn was due primarily to an increase in wages per patient day which rose by 16% per year and to a lesser extent to an increase in costs and usage of materials which rose by 8.9% per year.

In Quebec a lack of hospital beds does not seem to have been a serious restraint on hospital usage. Over the last 15 years they have been increased by 1.9% per thousand population and our hospitals in general do not have extensive waiting lists. One must conclude that the removal of economic restraints on hospital entry, surprisingly to some, has not caused excess usage. The impact of free hospitalization on hospitals and medical education has nevertheless been real but it has been indirect.

It has been the consequence of the prodigious increase in hospital costs to the state. They have risen 14.9% *per year* for the past

15 years in Quebec, and this is causing the state to be increasingly absorbed in the problem of economizing in expenditures in the health field. Professor Robert Evans of U.B.C. estimates that the expenditure of the Canadian citizen on personal health care has risen from 3½% to around 7% of his personal income between 1953 and 1971.

The state's ability to achieve restraint in further increases in the face of unionization of all health personnel including nurses, residents and interns is at this time problematical. The danger to medical schools is that it may be found easier to cut spending on items like medical education and medical research. An index that this danger is real is the budget of the Canadian Medical Research Council which has been increased by only 5% per annum over the past 5 years.

State expenditure on health took a further rise with universal medicare which came to our country around 1970. Here it is much harder to find precise information as to whether this caused an excess use requiring additional restraints. Most information is contained in a series of excellent studies conducted in Montreal the year before and for two years following the introduction of Medicare by Enterline and Corbett and Allison MacDonald and their colleagues. (1973)

They found that the average waiting time for a doctor's appointment increased from 6 to 11 days between 1969 and 1972. This was, however, not entirely due to the feared abuse of the system since they also found a reduction of 8½ hours in the average physician's working week (54.8 to 43.6). There were also changes in the pattern of patient contact. There was a fall in telephone contact (unremunerated in the present fee tariff), in home visits and hospital visits (relatively poorly remunerated) and an increase in office visits which are relatively better remunerated. At the same time there was a marked shift of services from persons in upper to lower income groups.

These studies suggest that abuse of the system has not been great and that increased service has been provided to lower income groups where it was previously relatively deficient. However, they do suggest that the method of remuneration may be having considerable effects on the nature of medical practice. Economic factors rather than health needs may in future increasingly influence such items as the use of laboratory tests and the time spent in interviewing and examining a patient. In so far as this is wasteful or contrary to optimal medical care these factors must be defined and analysed so that they may be countered where necessary. Here is an unorthodox form of research in which our medical schools will become increasingly involved in future years.

I will now briefly turn to the question of medical student enrollment and consider in what ways this is influencing the medical schools. It is only fifteen years since Canada's medical schools were concerned about the small number of applicants for medicine and some schools had difficulty in filling their first year classes. Since then however, the situation has changed radically.

In the last ten years our schools have expanded their enrollment and four new schools have been opened and openings for incoming students have been increased by 83%. In spite of this, however, the situation in the medical schools has changed from one of a shortage of good applicants to one of tremendous excess. For example in 1972 according to Collishaw and Grainger (1972) there were across Canada 6.2 applicants for each available place. It is my impression that this pressure to enter medicine has increased even further in the subsequent two years. For example, this year to select an incoming class of 160 my own school has had to consider 2,400 applications.

The reason for this pressure can be the subject of speculation. Very little is due to population growth which has gone up 1.8% per year over the past 15 years. More may be due to rising levels of affluence in the population. A cynic might tend to relate the most recent increase to the increase in physician's earnings which have resulted from Medicare.

Thus Professor R. Evans tells us that the change in physician's net earnings in Quebec from 1969 to 1971, the years spanning the introduction of universal Medicare in our province, was 51%. There was of course, an increase in all salaries and wages over the same period which he estimates at 15.6% but it is clear that the relative income status of physicians has risen very dramatically following Medicare legislation.

I personally suspect that the recent pressure to enter medicine is also due to a substantial but unmeasurable dissatisfaction with alternate career choices such as business, law, engineering, etc. and a restriction in career opportunities in science. The idea of a life of service and of healing is attractive to our young people. This, with scientific interest and the certainty of status and relative affluence adds up to an attraction to the medical career which is irresistible.

But what should we in the medical schools do about it? In a free enterprise system the schools would expand until all the students who could pay were satisfied or until all the patients who could afford one had a doctor. There would be a glut.

In a fully socialist society like China there would again be no problem for a medical school. The need for health workers of each type would be identified and the medical schools would produce the required number of doctors who would then proceed to where they were needed.

But we are operating what is virtually a nationalized service in the context of a free enterprise system. The onus is on someone to make an attempt to define the need and to adjust our schools to meet it. This is clearly not a task for medical schools alone.

To make any sense this will have to be applied at the national level, indeed there will need to be international involvement since movement of medical manpower is relatively free and in Canada around half of our Medical profession presently comes in already trained from foreign lands.

Our governments have tended to make the problem for the medical schools somewhat harder by their changing perceptions of needs. Until about 6 months ago, I would have said our politicians were responding primarily to the public's demands for more personal physicians. Thus we have been encouraged to expand our schools and to accentuate residency training in family medicine. In Quebec the licensing body has been encouraged to facilitate the licensing of foreign doctors.

But the mounting costs of the health service and the suspicion that doctors create their own demand is starting to cause second thoughts. We already have twenty per cent more doctors per head of population as England has and it would seem that our Government is beginning to wonder if our higher costs haven't maybe got something to do with this.

The sort of information behind this thinking comes from studies such as that of Professor Vayda of McMaster University (1973). He has recently compared the prevalence of surgeons and surgery in England and Wales and in Canada. In Canada there are not only 1.4 times as many surgeons per head of population as in England and Wales but a good deal of surgery is still carried out by general practitioners. The prevalence of those who use the knife is thus far higher as are the rates for certain forms of surgery. Vayda found that while the age standardized rates for appendectomy were very comparable in our two countries the rates for elective and discretionary procedures such as adenoidectomy, hemorrhoidectomy and inguinal herniorraphy were two or more times higher in Canada. The rate of cholecystectomy is 7 times higher in Canada.

From data such as these, health administrators are liable to conclude that doctors create their own demands and that the right way to check spiraling health costs is to limit the number of physicians. There is of course an alternate method. Vayda also points out that in those populations who are covered by prepaid schemes there is no direct financial gain involved in the procedure,

the incidence of these operations in North America is very comparable to Britain. However in Canada there are very powerful pressures
to retain the fee-for-service principle and it seems more likely at
this time that our Governments will not attempt to develop capitation formulae but will instead restrain the increase in the number of
practicing physicians.

We have not been told to cut back on the enrollment of medical
students. However, in Quebec we have been instructed within the
last few months to restrict the enrollment of foreign graduates in
our Residency training programs to 15%. Since a year of Residency
training is mandatory for most immigrant physicians this will substantially reduce the input of immigrants into our provincial health
system which at the present time is around 45% of the total.

There is danger to our medical schools and to medical education
in these swings of policy. The greatest is that, applied by the
massive hand of the state, they may affect all schools equally. In
doing so they must tend to make all schools more equal, to diminish
the ability to differentiate and to experiment. During the 'Research
Era' all schools tended to mimic the Harvard model and have their
own electron probes and computer installations lest they forego the
tremendous financial and other gifts that went with medical research.

The more recent incentives to produce more primary physicians
at a faster rate also applies to all schools. They are resulting in
renewed initiatives in family practice training, in a reduction in
the duration of medical training and especially basic science training,
not just in some schools but in all. I believe rather, that what we
should be aiming for is further differentiation of training patterns,
not standardization.

In conclusion, the health legislation introduced in our country
in recent years is indeed having significant effects on medical schools,
on hospitals and on clinical teachers. These effects are complex and
since there is no simple or single solution to the problem which this
legislation has created it is appropriate that schools should be
encouraged to experiment and to differentiate.

Thus, to train our medical scientists, our medical innovators, we
will always need true university type schools where scientific
training is given in depth and where biological research is of excellence. But not all schools need compete in this form of excellence.
We also will need schools whose primary role is to produce physicians,
in particular primary care physicians and in large enough numbers
to fulfil society's needs. I submit that we should not attempt to
force all schools into this primary training role but should be clear
that we need at least two quite different types of medical schools
in the future.

These two types of schools will differ in the sort of students they select, in the nature of their curricula and in their length. To those who object that this will 'produce two classes of doctors' I must say that I fully concur. It is high time we produced two or more classes. One does not train all aeronautical engineers to fly aeroplanes nor need all pilots be trained in the theory of aeronautical engineering.

In spite of Flexner, it is surely not necessary to make every primary physician an in-depth health scientist nor every medical school a center of biomedical research. To fulfil society's needs both in university education and in health manpower training we must experiment and develop schools with clearer role definitions. This has been made more urgent by society's decision to supply health care to all. The alternative to such differentiation is homogeneity, the development of an all purpose medical school where primary physician training will be inappropriate, selection of students for future roles inept, and where medical science itself will flounder.

References

1. McDonald, A. D., McDonald, J. C., Steinmetz, N., Enterline, P. E., and Salter, V. (1973) *Medical Care* 11, 269-286.
2. Enterline, P. E., McDonald, J. C., McDonald, A. D., Davignon, L., and Salter, V. (1973) New Eng. J. Med. 288, 1152-1155.
3. Enterline, P. E., Salter, V., McDonald, A. D., and McDonald, J. C. (1973) New Eng. J. Med. 289, 1174-1178.
4. Collishaw, N. E., and Grainger, P. M. (1972) Canad. Med. Assoc. J. 106, 153.
5. Vayda, E. (1973). New Eng. J. Med. 289, 1224-1229.

Chapter 9

PROVISION OF HEALTH CARE IN THE COMMUNITY—
THE EXPERIENCE IN HAMILTON, ONTARIO, SINCE 1965

J. HAY
McMaster University, Hamilton, Ontario, Canada

PROVISION OF health care at the community level is one aspect of the global challenge to resolve the world's health care problems and it is this aspect that I invite you to consider. In discussing health care, a distinction should be made between the health status of the population and the actual organization and delivery of health care. It is the latter we will be concerned with here.

To move from the general to the specific, I would like first to identify some conflicts and deficiencies in the Canadian health care system and then to focus on these in the context of the city and district of Hamilton, in the Province of Ontario, the general goal being to show how this community has tried to rationalize the organization and provision of health services.

In Canada the provision of personal health services is a matter of provincial jurisdiction. The provinces, with federal financial assistance, have established universal pre-paid health services that have virtually removed financial barriers to medical and hospital care. The Ontario Health Insurance Plan, for instance, 'provides insurance through premium payment to the Plan. Premium-free insurance is available to those with no taxable income and to all residents aged 65 years and over; 50% premium assistance is available to other low-income persons. The scheme covers almost all residents of Ontario and its coverage extends outside the province and outside Canada.'

The general level of health services in a country can be measured in terms of three overall indicators—the ratio of various health professions to the population, the ratio of treatment facilities to the population, and the extent of pre-paid insurance coverage. Using these indicators, Table 1 shows how Canada compares with some other countries.

'In hospital and medical insurance coverage, Canada equals the best of the five countries chosen for comparison; it leads in respect of physicians, is in the middle rank in respect of hospital beds and is second only to Australia in nurses. Since the countries chosen are among those with the best health care services in the world, there

Table 1

Country	% covered by Medical and Hospital Insurance	No. of Hosp. beds per 10,000 Population	No. of Physicians per 10,000 Population	No. of Nurses per 10,000 Population
Australia	79% (Hosp.) 75% (Med.)	117.4	11.8	66.6
Canada	Almost 100%	102.3	15.7	57.3
Denmark	96.7%	89.4	14.5	53.4
Sweden	Almost 100%	145.8	12.4	43.7
United Kingdom	Almost 100%	111.4	12.5	35.1
United States	85% (Hosp.) 65% (Reg. Med.) 35% (Maj. Med.)	82.7	15.3	49.2

is no doubt that ... Canada is among the world leaders.' (New Perspectives of the Health of Canadians.)

This having been said, it must be added that the introduction of universal health insurance has not, of itself, raised the level of health of the population. Furthermore, the existence of a number of conflicting goals within the health system has given rise to some very basic problems.

On the one hand, for instance, it is a goal to make physician services equally accessible to everyone; on the other hand, in a free enterprise system, it is a goal that physicians should be permitted to practise where they wish and, within broad limits, how they wish in terms of the range of services and continuity of care provided. Other goal conflicts involve the right of ready access to health care as against the freedom of physicians to select their specific field of training; the logic of services being provided by personnel trained only to the level of skill needed as against the practice of physicians and dentists of carrying out tasks that could be done as well or better by others at less cost; and finally, the general agreement of a need for more research into the nature of health problems and for more effective prevention as against the disproportionate increase in energy and money spent treating existing illness.

Problems relating directly to these conflicts include an annual rate of cost escalation ranging on a national basis from 12% to 16%, which far exceeds the economic growth of the country; the concentration of specialty services in hospitals; the random distribution of physicians and variable quality of care without regard for community need; a lack of co-ordination between primary care, secondary care and other health services; and the inaccessibility of services in certain areas. In short, to quote the recent report of the Ontario Health Planning Task Force, 'no plan has been developed for the delivery of health services in relation to the overall needs of the population.'

The terms primary care and secondary care may deserve a word of explanation. In the present context and as defined by the Ontario Health Planning Task Force recently, primary care is the major health care sector. 'It is the first point of contact for the individual with the health care system ... and should provide services on a continuous basis. Secondary care is a resource to primary care (and provides services) to those who require more specialized care than is available in the primary sector.' A corollary is that the interface between primary and secondary care must permit continuity of service, regardless of where it is provided.

In this situation the challenge is to develop, on a voluntary basis if possible, a system for providing comprehensive health care to the population within the limits of available financial resources. The question is, how?

In Hamilton the approach has been through the integration of health services and education on a regional basis and a working partnership is emerging of the public, municipal, provincial and federal government, health professions, social agencies and educators. While the evolution of these arrangements has been neither painless nor easy, it is occurring and has become the hallmark, so to speak, of the local situation.

By way of background, Hamilton is a manufacturing city at the southwestern end of Lake Ontario. The population is 300,000; immediately adjacent Townships increase the population to over 500,000. The McMaster planning area which the Province of Ontario has recognized for purposes of health care and education contains 1,400,000 people. There are six hospitals in the Hamilton district, including the University Hospital, with a total of 3,500 beds. All these hospitals are actively involved in health education and regional planning. There are about 762 practising physicians in the city, of whom slightly less than one half are general practitioners (family physicians) and there is, for the most part, a clear distinction between general and specialty practice, in that most specialists confine themselves to referral practice.

Family physicians who so desire may have staff appointments at one or more hospitals, including the University Hospital, where they may admit and treat their patients, subject to rational checks and balances based on the experience and proven ability of the individual practitioner. They function as active medical staff members and participate as well by serving on various medical staff committees. Hospital practice is more attractive to some family physicians than to others and the degree of involvement varies considerably, but the choice is the family physician's and he may make the hospital side of his practice as major or as minor a part of his total activities as he wishes.

A significant feature of the medical scene in Hamilton is the Academy of Medicine, an active professional and educational organization that provides a forum for dialogue amongst the city's physicians and, in co-operation with the hospitals and the medical faculty, supports an active program of continuing education.

The School of Medicine at McMaster was established in 1965 with the appointment of Dr. John R. Evans as Dean and Vice-President of the Division of Health Sciences. The first class graduated in 1971 and the Health Sciences Centre was formally opened in 1972. A proposal has recently been approved by the University Senate to incorporate the School of Medicine and the School of Nursing into a Faculty of Health Science.

The concept of the regionalization of health services has been adopted by a number of countries and implemented in a variety of forms. In Canada, the report of a Royal Commission stated in 1964 (The Hall Report)—'Provision must be made at the local, regional, provincial and federal levels for representative Health Planning Councils to ensure democratic participation in the setting of goals and objectives and the meeting of human needs.' A federal task force in 1972 (The Hastings Report) proposed 'development by the provinces, in mutual agreement with public and professional groups, of a significant number of community health centres as non-profit corporate bodies in a fully integrated health services system.' An Ontario Task Force, in reviewing the Hastings Report the following year, endorsed local planning and development and proposed, among other things, an experimental approach through various groupings of health professionals and alternative methods of payment. This year an Ontario Health Planning Task Force urged (The Mustard Report) that health services should be organized on a regional basis as rapidly as possible and made quite specific suggestions as to how this should be done. The report also stressed the need to promote the development of the primary care sector, to ensure integration of primary and secondary care and for the evaluation of effectiveness at all levels.

Against this background it is interesting that in Hamilton the initiative in regionalization arose from within the community and antedated both the present degree of government involvement and the establishment of the Medical School at McMaster. Regionalization of health services began in Hamilton as an attempt to rationalize the hospital system. In the first instance this was initiated by agreement between the hospitals and led to the formation of the Hamilton District Council in 1965. All hospitals and the medical school were represented on this body, which was advisory both to the hospitals and government. The District Hospital Council was expanded in 1970 to a District Health Council with broad representation from many agencies and professional groups. Although the Council is advisory and acts by consensus, it is a very influential force in the development of health programs in the Hamilton region. For example, agreement has been reached that all proposals for capital construction involving new programs, regardless of cost, and for reconstruction of existing facilities where the cost exceeds $100,000 must be approved by the Council before any submission may be made to the provincial Ministry of Health for approval and funding.

While the Council is still somewhat hospital-dominated, the public is being encouraged to serve at all levels; the Chairman and Vice-Chairman, for example, are citizens who sit as concerned individuals and not as representatives of any institutions or groups. A pattern of organization is emerging voluntarily which does involve other health agencies, which increases citizen representation and participation and which will, it is hoped, eventually meet the needs of the local population and involve appropriately both the general public and the providers of health services (Evans, 1970).

Any co-operative venture of this sort makes demands on the participants, of which one of the most threatening is the giving up of some degree of autonomy. Progress is sometimes disappointingly slow but despite the difficulties, a number of tangible accomplishments have emerged through the district programs of the Health Council. For example, the Extended Care Program has developed an assessment and placement service to identify the extended care needs of the district and to assist health professionals in assessing the needs of their patients and placing them where these needs can best be met. This service has assisted in the assessment and placement of almost 5000 patients since the program was initiated in 1971.

An integrated District Program of Laboratory Medicine has been developed to meet the needs of patients receiving health care, not only in hospitals, but in other health facilities including doctors' offices. Through the program, the resources of the district hospitals, McMaster University and the provincial laboratory have been combined into a single laboratory service providing a complete range of high quality service without unnecessary duplication of staff and equipment. This program is now funded on a district, rather than an institutional basis, with its own administrative staff and is providing an economical, comprehensive program of laboratory services, as well as subserving the needs of the University, Mohawk

College and district hospitals for education, research and development in the field of Laboratory Medicine.

A Pharmacy Program has made possible the group purchasing of pharmaceuticals and hospital supplies with considerable saving to the participating institutions. This program has, in fact, been so popular that it has been joined by several hospitals in adjacent districts.

Other programs, at varying stages of development involve Alcoholism, Cardiovascular disease, Emergency Services, Nephrology, Neurosciences, Respirology and Rehabilitation Medicine.

A thorny problem facing the Council at this moment is the matter of bed closure. On a per capita basis there are too many hospital beds in Hamilton—partly as a legacy from the era of hospital autonomy and partly because the planning of the 1960's was based on five beds per thousand population rather than the current revised figure of four beds per thousand—and the Ministry of Health has indicated that over two hundred beds must be shut down. Proposals have been developed to centralize facilities in obstetrics and pediatrics as a means of adapting to the reduced number of beds and, by consolidation, of achieving greater efficiency and an improved quality of service. The issue, however, poses a major conflict of interests to the hospitals and the medical profession and its resolution will test the strength of local commitment to the integration of health services.

The Division of Health Sciences at McMaster has been, since its establishment in 1965, an active participant in the regional development of health services and education. The 'founding fathers' believed, and the provincial government heartily endorsed the view, that the faculty should avoid at all costs an ivory tower attitude and address itself, with others, to solving the practical problems of providing health care in the community.

With regard to the organization of the Division of Health Sciences, there was concern from the beginning to develop what the Dean referred to as an 'overriding sense of purpose and commitment to the objectives of the Health Sciences Centre as a whole' (Evans, 1970). Recognizing that the objectives 'are usually ill-defined and tend to be subordinated to the aspirations of individuals or to the goals of administrative sub-units' it was early determined that programs should be defined in terms of the objectives of the Division of Health Sciences and that the allocation of resources should be to programs rather than to academic departments. This principle has, in fact, been applied.

Reflecting the faculty's concern with the provision of primary care in the community and the need to develop a more balanced system of primary and secondary care, one of the first programs to be established, in 1967, was a three-year postgraduate program in Family Medicine. The assumption was that physicians who selected Family Medicine as a career and who were well prepared for the role would be more effective and efficient in providing primary care than physicians whose education may not have been appropriate to primary care or whose professional interests might lie elsewhere.

While Family Medicine may not be, in all circumstances, the only or best modality for providing primary care, it is recognized as such for Ontario in a recent policy statement by the provincial government to the effect that 50% of the province's medical graduates shall enter postgraduate programs in Family Medicine and that not more than 50% shall enter the other specialties. The numbers and quality of applicants to the McMaster Postgraduate Program in Family Medicine suggest that this is a realistic way, in this community, of increasing the number of physicians with a professional interest and appropriate training in primary care. We are currently taking about 30 residents per year into the Postgraduate Program in Family Medicine and about 80 into the other specialty programs.

It should be stressed that this program is not solely the responsibility of the Department of Family Medicine but of the Faculty as a whole. The other specialties are substantially involved, not only in the program in family medicine but in the development of a full range of primary care services, including emergency services, and the establishment of an effective interface between the primary and secondary levels of care.

Parenthetically, one of the most exciting developments has been the increasingly extensive educational involvement of practising physicians. For example, in addition to the 21 full-time faculty physicians in the Department of Family Medicine, over 70 family physicians in the Hamilton district teach in student electives, the clinical clerkship and the residency program. This is particularly significant in that it represents a positive resolution of an initially difficult town/gown situation and while it may seem peripheral to the issue of community health care, it is actually quite central, indicating a willingness on the part of the profession to accept new responsibilities and a redefinition of roles in the health care system.

The logic of primary care being provided by professionals other than physicians has been widely recognized as a means of improving the accessibility of care in an economical way. Since, in Canada, the nurse is seen as the professional best able to assume a broader role and to supplant physician care in certain circumstances, a Nurse Practitioner Program was established by McMaster in 1971, operated jointly by the Schools of Nursing and Medicine and funded by the Ontario Ministry of Health.

The key educational principles of the program were:

1. The orientation of the curriculum should emphasize the nurse's development of added skills and clinical problem solving. An orientation that is primarily procedural is undesirable.
2. To develop nurse practitioners in an apprentice system would handicap assessment of the nurse's performance and might impair the evolution of desirable patterns of practice. Therefore the education of nurse practitioners should take place in post-secondary institutions.
3. The program should be interdisciplinary. Faculties of Medicine and Nursing should be jointly deployed; nurses should learn new skills together with physicians who are learning new roles.

The criteria for admission of a nurse to the program were:

1. Current registration with the College of Nurses of Ontario.
2. Employment in the office of a family physician or in a family health care centre.
3. Participation of the associated physician in the program.

Priority was given to residents of under-serviced areas who undertook to return to such localities.

The program was funded initially for a three-year period and it is expected to provide for the education of over 100 nurse practitioners during that time. 'Preliminary indicators of satisfaction, acceptance and financial viability suggested these programs will effectively serve important health care expectations of the population' (Spitzer & Kergin, 1973).

In keeping with the philosophy of development programs in education and service that respond to the needs of the community a project known as the Northwestern Ontario Medical Program (NOMP) was initiated in 1972. While the program is not designed to meet community needs in Hamilton district, it does involve a number of health professionals and administrators at McMaster and is included here as an example of effective co-operation between faculty, practising physicians, the provincial government and local communities in attacking a specific set of health care problems.

The ultimate goal of the program is better health care for the people of the Northwestern part of the Province of Ontario, an area of over 200,000 square miles with a population of about 225,000 people, of whom one half are in the city of Thunder Bay. The terrain is rough, the climate is harsh and except for Thunder Bay and some of the larger towns, health services could be described as less than adequate. Medical students are selected from that area by the same criteria as other student applicants. They, with other students, can spend periods in teaching practices in the area, both as undergraduates and residents, undergraduates on an elective basis and the residents on a three-month rotation in their second or third year. In addition, attachments are available for students to specialists and specialty services in Thunder Bay. This program is extremely popular with students and residents, while the local physicians, of whom about 45 are involved, report a keen sense of professional enrichment. This is perhaps one of the most powerful approaches to continuing education that has been developed in any of our programs.

Success will depend primarily on an effective working relationship between the physician teachers and the faculty, a relationship made more difficult by the thousand miles that separate them. A contractual arrangement has been developed on a partnership basis between the faculty and the Thunder Bay Medical Society that involves continuing close liaison between the two groups, frequent site visits, periodic workshop meetings and an extensive built-in evaluation component. The program is financed by the Ontario Ministry of Health.

While it is fair to say that some progress has been made, obviously a great deal remains to be done. Prerequisites for the success of a regionally integrated programmatic approach include a number of difficult role changes for all concerned. The public must participate more directly through membership on planning boards, for instance. The provincial and federal governments must be prepared to allocate executive authority and adequate funds to the district health councils. The hospitals must rethink their function with respect, for example, to greater outreach into the community and the provision of more comprehensive ambulatory services. Health professions must assume a greater share of the joint responsibility for organization and administration of the health care system, including experimentation with models such as the Community Health Centre. Social agencies must submerge their individual aspirations, where necessary, in the interests of the effective co-operative endeavour. Educators must assume responsibility for the development of innovative programs in health care and education (and in this context the two are inseparable) that relate to community needs, as well as for health care research that will permit fine tuning of the system, as it were, over time.

To recapitulate, I have tried, however briefly, to indicate how one community through an integrated approach, is attempting to resolve some principal issues in the provision of health care. The point has been made that health services, education and research in Hamilton are highly co-ordinated, at least by Canadian standards, at the district level and examples have been given of specific programs to illustrate this. The willingness of institutions and individuals to desert traditional roles and assume new responsibilities, in spite of manifest conflicts, has been identified. Finally, reference has been made to some of the prerequisites of success in the development of programs whose ultimate goal is an effective response to community needs.

Chapter 10

DOES THE FRENCH MEDICAL CARE SYSTEM MEET THE
NEEDS OF THE POPULATION AND SATISFY
THE PHYSICIANS?

J. C. SOURNIA
Service Médical de l'Assurance Maladie, Paris, France

A RECENT working group of the WHO enumerated the different
aspects attempting to measure the value of a health care system,
and I shall examine some of these criteria with respect to the
French medical care system, but two aspects are generally minimized.

The first one is chronological: the working of a system can only
be estimated over several years and during this time neither the
medical technique, nor the system, remain stationary. Every estimation is thus more or less mistaken and it would be illusive to try to
consider the comparative morbidity statistics bound to particular
sanitary measures, or to cost-efficacy calculations, as having a too
high mathematical precision.

The second one is psychological: the WHO considered 'the
degree of service adequacy' to the needs of the population, as well
as the 'acceptability of services' by the population and I shall develop
these points; but it did not mention the nevertheless essential
adhesion of the medical profession to the system. If the needs of
one party and the wants of the other are not supplied, other kinds
of medicine develop outside the system and elements of the system
are either nonemployed or overemployed, thus diminishing its
efficiency and performance. Its value has to be considered from the
point of view of the population taken care of and the one of the
professions taking care of it.

Evaluation of the medical care on the sick of the population

General mortality and morbidity of the nation are the simplest
judgment criteria for the good medical care of a population. Life
expectancy in France is the same as in other similarly developed
countries, where the medical care system is more authoritative,
possesses higher resources, or applies to a lower population. Infectious
diseases practically disappeared, the last poliomyelitic vaccine led to
the eradication of the illness. Mortality connected with birth

problems (mortality of the mother, morti-natality, child morbidity) is higher than expected, but diminishes regularly.

Tuberculosis has changed in a few decades thanks to the use of antibiotics and BCG vaccination. Tuberculosis of the serosa (peritoneum, pleura, articulations) disappeared; some bone tuberculosis still exists, lung lesions are only observed among Mediterranean or African migrant workers; neither sanitary controls in the native country before leaving for France, nor medical examinations in France before recruiting are totally effective, consequently this disease still prevails among the immigrated people and retains a certain contagiousness for the autochthonous population. France gradually suppresses the systematic chest X-ray services because of their feeble output (0.6 cases tracked down for 1000 exposures).

The struggle against cancer and cardiovascular diseases is at the same point as in the other European countries, the results being uncertain with respect to their cause.

The financial yield of the system, that is the relation between the obtained results and the spent resources, is difficult to establish and the countries all over the world meet the same lack of precision in this field. It is possible to compare the cost and the yields of two therapeutic methods, for instance hemodialysis for the treatment of chronic renal insufficiency, as used in a treatment centre or at the patient's home; but it is much more difficult to compare the expenses of a medical care system and its results on population morbidity with what would happen if it were not applied to a population having the same number of persons, same setting of age, same kind of profession, of life, etc. . . .

I shall mention three kinds of expenses the yield for which France is questioning.

In France as well as in a certain number of European countries, pharmacopoeia progress, its innovations and efficiency are accompanied by passionate reactions from different social or political classes. Physicians are said to have too many drugs at their disposal, the latter being manufactured at too high expenses by the captains of industry and sold at too high prices by the pharmacists. It is known that certain states adopted these widely held opinions and took action accordingly. The French Sickness Insurance spent 8.6 milliards F.F. during the last year and besides, the population bought medicines for 5 milliards F.F., without a medical prescription, excluding cosmetics, beauty preparations, or current medicines sold without prescription. We try by means of education to slow down this mostly useless and certainly harmful automedication. We also try to limit collectivity expenses to the sole repayment of the scientifically adequate drugs, meaning that the number of repaid products should diminish. As for the drugs price, it will only be lowered by means of international agreements regulating raw materials prices, moralizing the industrial patents system and regulating the successive royalty processes: these wishes are, in the present state of world trade, only utopias.

France also examines the yield of its medical care establishments, the two third of beds of which are public and one third private. The Sickness Insurance in 1973 spent 42.6 milliards for medical care, 19.5 milliards of which being paid to public and private hospitals. Could the same medical care be offered at less expense? Are the hospital manpower and material equipments employed to the maximum of their possibilities? Are our equipments well distributed inside the country? Is the medical care better and less expensive at the hospital than outside the hospital? The sums spent on hospital care become so important that we will not watch unconcerned their continuous increase; we consider new distributions inside the hospital between medical care with or without hospital stay, and between medical care inside or outside hospital institution; we also try to work out new management methods that would better account for the cost-profit yields of the hospital. These management problems are the concern of the majority of western countries.

A third preoccupation is due to the organization and expenses related to biology and especially biochemistry. In a few years biochemical investigations became the essential supports of every medical diagnosis and the checking tools for every hormonal, surgical or other medicamentous therapy. The extraordinary increase of investigations consumption was also multiplied by the evolution of auto-analyzers, allowing quicker, less expensive and safer examinations.

Are all the examinations asked for by the physicians, or the patients necessary? Of course not; we know it, but how can we prove it? Even if the cost of an investigation is of only a few francs, even if it is integrated to an auto-analyzer chain, it represents a useless expenditure if it is not necessary to affirm the diagnosis or to check the treatment; at the same time the apparatus with increasingly better performances are increasingly expensive and are only paid off with certain consumption. In this field also the national equipment must be co-ordinated, planned, for a better management and an optimum efficiency.

Introducing financial or book-keeping data to medicine is difficult due to the treated matter comprising many subcategories and to the opposed misunderstandings of physicians and administrators. Anyway the expenses increase every year and we have to know better the expense items in order to check them with a better precision.

The French system can be considered as a success because of the easy accessibility to medical care. From the economical point of view the medical care is not completely free of charge because, depending on the case, the Sickness Insurance refunds 70% or 100% of the expenses. Long and expensive diseases are totally refunded. The Insurance gives also daily allowances for the insured people that have to stop their work, the allowances being calculated according to the usual salary. We still have to progress because short and mild diseases, with a 20% or 30% participation for medical prescriptions or biological, or radiological investigations, represent a burden for low salary families.

Socially, all the inhabitants of France, citizens or not, working or not, have a right to be protected against diseases; this is true, of course, also for the foreign workers and their families. Nevertheless a disfavoured area of 2% persists, concerning mainly old people that never had a salaried activity since the generalization of social security; but it continuously diminishes thanks to special measures taken in this field.

Geographically one can admit that all the sick persons of France can find near their home either the physician, or the medical care institution they need, thanks to two particular phenomena.

To begin with, in France we still have general practitioners 25,800 for a total of 70,000 physicians; thus, besides the hospitals the general practitioners receive the patients at their office, or go to visit them at home; this avoids queuing up at the hospital.

Then, our medical equipments are rather equally distributed along the territory; we try to correct the remaining technical disparities (modernizing out-of-date equipment, overequipped installations, neighbouring underequipped ones) by means of a planning more or less well accepted by the promoters and the physicians.

We may congratulate ourselves on the good accessibility of services, without forgetting that the system has to be supervised in order to keep its balance.

What are the conclusions with respect to meeting the needs of the population? First of all the idea of 'need' has to be defined. If one considers the 'objective' needs as they can be defined by the epidemiologists, the practising physicians or the administrators responsible for public health, the system still offers obvious gaps. Besides the already mentioned imperfections, one has to evoke all kinds of handicapped people, adults or children, with sensorial, motorial, psychic, or psychomotorial infirmities. Our French society is still hard for them and their families and the aid they are receiving by means of resources, housing, education, socio-affective comfort is quite inadequate. The same applies to aged people, especially if they are poor; they have been kept for centuries in never modernized asylums and they do not accept this segregation any longer. Yet maintaining handicapped as well as aged people at home creates still unsolved problems.

As for the 'subjective' needs, as they are rightly or wrongly experienced by the population, they seem to be correctly satisfied, even if we know that ignorance in the sanitary field lessens the demands. In any case, during electoral episodes people do not talk much about health in France and, as a rule, the French population considers itself in good health.

Despite the information efforts of the physicians, neither the public authorities nor the population are very keen on taking steps to diminish the damages of well known plagues like: overnourishment, alcohol, tobacco, traffic accidents. Prevention in these fields would represent the most efficient medical action, but it does not touch the collectivity and consequently no political step is taken against them.

People are less interested in the cost of medical care or equipment, as well as in the training of the medical and paramedical professions, than in the safety of medical care (if people die under surgery many newspapers articles write about it, but so far very few law actions are brought) and especially as they insist upon receiving pleasant medical care. This last item inspires controversies concerning the lack of comfort of certain institutions, the telephone missing, the visiting hours; 'humanizing the hospitals' is the program of the successive Ministers. Nevertheless the French medical system is adequate in this field also, thanks to the coexistence of two kinds of hospital care: either in public institutions (371,000 beds), or in private institutions (161,000 beds). The population is sure to find the necessary technical competence of practising physicians and the best medical care safety in the great public hospitals, as well as a better comfort and pleasant care in smaller private clinics. The ideal of course, would be to find safety and pleasant care at the same place, but the two things are expensive! In any case this variety in medical care distribution suits the public, and the competition between public and private sectors is fruitful.

The conclusion: as a whole, the subjective or objective sanitary needs of the population are correctly satisfied.

The French Health care system evaluated by the physicians

The medical care distribution system to the nation was elaborated along a history of one century and a half; the public noticed it only inasmuch as the families' financial charges became gradually less important. On the contrary the medical profession was more susceptible to an evolution that transformed a completely liberal profession, relating to crafts, into one having to submit to a fees tariffing and to an administrative organization becoming gradually heavier with the considerable increase of the concerned sums.

This explains the continuous restlessness of the physicians, which is not particular to France. The officials responsible for the public health of a country cannot consider the physicians' ill-humour merely as hard-to-please children's whims; because this provokes (the experience of several countries proves it) the development of parallel or underhand medical practices or also of charlatanism of all kinds. Finally the population is not taken care of according to the medical care system, the system fails.

1. Among 70,000 physicians practising in France, 49,100 practise their profession partially or completely in the 'liberal' manner, medical attendance being paid according to a fee for service tariff established by an agreement between the medical unions and the social security. The physicians did not accept easily the tariffing of their fees, they hated the very idea of it for a long time; nowadays it forced itself upon them, but 19% of them have the possibility, based on academic titles accepted by their colleagues, to charge higher fees. The tariff is regularly kept up to date by bilateral negotiations twice a year. This system is already applied for several years and satisfies both parties; the medical fees represent only 17% of the nation's total health expenditure and the physicians consider their income as satisfactory.

Nevertheless neither society nor the physicians are stable and distortions in income level and way of life, are taking place, alarming for the future because they are prejudicial to the acceptance of the system by the physicians.

They note that their income increases less than inflation. This phenomenon is not peculiar to the profession, seeing that during inflation the salaries fixed by the more or less official intervention of the state are always lower than the real cost of life. But thus a difference establishes itself between the liberal practice physicians and the salaried ones : the latter increase in number (hospital and/ or universitary physicians, public health, factory, school, Sickness Insurance physicians, etc ...) and they are essential to the country's medical well-being.

2. On the other hand France is very keen on keeping the family doctors in the medical care system. For the public they represent a considerable safety element, being permanently at their disposal, having good general medical knowledge and being good counsellors for all problems of health hygiene, nutrition, etc.... They contribute to the acceptability of the medical care system and are also a factor for its good economical utilization, because a medical visit, or consultation is less expensive than losing a day to wait at the hospital, or even than hospitalization. These general practitioners' rough mean yearly income is of about 142,800 F. But these physicians have very tiring work because of the number of consulting hours, the intensity, rhythm, emergencies; they also have professional expenses. On the technical level some of them are dissatisfied by their job of 'first sorting out'. The drawbacks of this life are highest for the country physicians, whereas those in town have a more comfortable life, their wives and children have larger educational and cultural possibilities.

The general practioners found a remedy to these constraints by association in groups of three or four: thus, they can organize duty days and vacations in rotation and have in common certain staff, as well as professional equipments. This formula is developing slowly, the government and the Sickness Insurance encourage it and could even finance its development, but until now the physicians were too eager on independence to accept this offer. Group medicine is a kind of exercise upon which we rely very much in order to keep the family physicians we need in France. In fact their reduction would contribute to increase the importance of the medical care in hospitals with regard to the one in medical offices, a thing we do not want, and to lessen the medical care accessibility, which is sufficient for the time being.

Should the profession of general practitioner become less attractive for the physicians, the ratio of specialists would increase and this has to be avoided for several reasons. At present we count 23,200 specialists in France against 25,800 general practitioners. Contrary to the habit of other countries, the patients consult the specialist either on their own initiative, or at the advice of a general practitioner. The specialists often have a higher income than the general practitioners (212,000 F.F. rough mean yearly income), but this is not the rule. The basic difference attracting students toward specialization is the way of life. The specialist generally lives in a middle sized town, is not disturbed at night or on Sundays, enjoys some leisure, a steadier family life and finds it easier to keep a satisfactory medical formation level. His superiority dwells more in his pleasant way of life than in the earned money.

The specialists' increase in number would extend the mean duration of medical studies, rendering them even more expensive to the collectivity; and people would have to undergo several specialists visits for the majority of simple medical diagnosis events, instead of a single, sufficient visit to the general practitioner. The dispensed medical care would cost more and be of lower quality.

After evoking the distortion between general practitioners and specialists, I have to mention also those existing among the specialists, always for the same reason: the way of life, the amount of the income, or both. Thus, from now on, there is a shortage in certain areas: students are no longer interested in dermatology because of the lack of patients, they avoid gynecology, obstetrics and anaesthesia because of too important professional obligations. These phenomena have bad consequences for the population: anaesthesia is given by hospital attendants the competence of which is suitable only to benign surgery, obstetrics is directed by physicians insufficiently formed for high risk pregnancies.

Changes in the distribution of the different kinds of medical care inside the sanitary system are observed, and these transformations are alarming for its good functioning, as well as for the quality of medicine. These tendencies could only be rectified by an authoritative proportioning of general practitioners and specialists, as well as by a planned and compulsory distribution of specialists between their different specialities and the different areas of the country. Only this planning would fit to a good management, but it does not belong to national traditions and would go against the fierce individualism of the physicians.

3. This is not the place for a psychological analysis of the medical profession, the declared claims of the associations, trade unions or orders being generally different from the hopes and determinations of physicians as individuals: every nation breeds physicians reflecting the mentality of the population, and all our occidental nations have the same difficulties to get particularistic individuals like physicians, professionally convinced of the individuality of human beings, into progressively constraining organizations and regulations.

How can we not be astounded in France at the contradictory preoccupations expressed by the physicians?

For a long time they defended the freedom of fees, they now discover that tariffing and social security avoid the unpaid bills and have suppressed the former medical proletariate of the working suburbs and the country-side.

They declare being attached to the fee for service system, nevertheless many of them are looking for salaried activities, at least for a part-time job.

They want to preserve the historically 'liberal' (this adjective allowing controversial definitions), that is free and independent, character of their profession, but they also want the state to insure the level of their income, they want security of work meaning a certain professional activity, they want sickness insurance, a prosperous pension. Their demands are those of the great trade unions fifty years ago, with at the same time an income level of the well-doing middle class and the professional freedom of the medieval craftsman. They are simultaneously contradictory and anachronistic, but one cannot neglect them because they are presented with skill and obstinacy sometimes with the support of the public; the latter being rid of the disease expense worries, keeps a religious respect for his physicians.

One can understand the anxiety of the officials for the medical care system of the country, its organization and financing. They know the obvious management errors, for instance in the functioning of the public and private medical care institutions and they know that collectivity resources cannot assume much longer the progressive increase of health expenses. But, at the same time, they are aware of the role of the medical profession concerning certain costly prescriptions not always absolutely necessary to the patient's health, the uselessly repeated biological analyses and radiological investigations, the too easily prescribed or prolonged hospital care: the good functioning of a medical care system presumes the understanding and active participation of the physicians managing it, that is the satisfaction of their desires compatible with the common interests.

Concerning the physicians, the government's task is to satisfy their rightful care about the moral protection due to the patient, their understandable anxiety for a sufficient remuneration, while laying upon them the obligation of social and economical constraints of modern medicine.

These requirements are not easy to conciliate, and without knowing the direction of the future French health system evolution, one may foresee deep changes for the coming years.

Chapter 11

THE PROVISION OF MEDICAL CARE AND ITS EFFECT ON EDUCATION IN FRANCE

J. SAMAILLE
Institut Pasteur de Lille

As PROFESSOR SOURNIA has explained, the French system of medical care seems at present to give satisfaction at the same time to physicians and to the population. But this satisfaction is the result of expenses which are pressurising more and more the national income.

The social budget* of the nation, meaning the whole of the procedures relative to various subscriptions, represent a total of 264 billions of francs for the year of 1974, being a little more than the State's budget, which totals a sum of 225 billions for that same year. Out of this budget of 264 Billions, 80% come from subscriptions on salaries. The charge of the social security system is nearly 50% of the total mass of salaries.

From 1973 to 1974 the rise has been of about 13,56% as far as subscriptions are concerned and of 15,81% for the expenses.

On this budget, 24%, that is 64 billion francs, concerns the sickness insurance (that is 25 B for hospitalisation, 13 B for home services, 12 B for prescriptions). The progression of these expenses may be appreciated when it is known that the cost of the sickness insurance has nearly doubled between 1969 and 1973.

During these last 20 years the growth rate has been of 14,8% against 10% for the whole of the national gross product.

Today the social budget represents 23% of the national gross product and sickness insurance 5,6%. We may wonder if such a growth will be tolerable in a context of economical crisis.

The whole of these activities is taken care of by a manpower which in 1968 could be estimated to 850,000 people, about 4,25% of the total active population. The provision of medical care employs a part of manpower practically identical to the one engaged in education. The progression appears to have been very quick, of about 5,2% per year between 1962 and 1968. Between 1968 and 1974, the annual rise of the health manpower has varied between

---

* The social budget concerns sickness insurance, pensions, family allowances, unemployment insurance, occupation casuality, housing allowances. Figures given here concern the budget of 1974 while SOURNIA's are those of 1973.

3,5 and 5%. We do not have at present precise figures but it
seems as if more than one million people are involved in 1973 in
health activities, which exceeds the number of people employed
in the Ministry of Education considered, as it is a single institution,
as the most important French enterprise and whose budget (57 B
in 1974) exceeds the 41,6 B of the budget of national defense.

The level of qualification of health manpower is higher than the
national average. Near 35% of employees that is more than 330,000
in 1973 have received a specialised sanitary education that is:

   70,000 physicians, with a density of 136 for 100,000
   23,000 dentists
    9,000 midwives
   18,000 pharmacists
  210,000 nurses and other technicians of health such as orthopho-
          nists and so on.

Among all this category of personnel the percentage of management is high. It is evidently the case for liberal professions:
physicians represent 71% of people in medical cabinet and dentists
63%. Nurses in the liberal system profess practically without help.
Proportion of management is also striking in pharmaceutical management where workers represent only 43% of the total. The case of
public hospitals is more complex; management and full time
physicians represent 5,7% of the total, technicians and nurses 24,6%.

It is evident that such an increase in the development of medical
care and medical staff may not have been without influence on the
system of medical education.

Regulation of the number of students

Knowing the level of qualifications of health personnel it is useful
to compare the number of students in this field with the total
figure in universities.

The number of medical students has abruptly increased from
45,800 in 1966 to more than 100,000 in 1969. The direct cause of
this growth is in fact the progression of the percentage of A level
students going to medical schools which was of 9,8% in 1963 and
rose to 12,8% in 1969. It is evident that such a sudden flow to the
medical schools is partly due to the relatively comfortable wages in
medical profession in France and also to the public's conviction that
medical consumption would be necessarily growing indefinitely.
In 1973, the total number of medical students remains the same as
in 1969, that is: 102,000 students divided in seven years of studies.

This stabilisation is due to the decision taken by public power in 1973 to limit to 8,200 the number of entries in the second year of medicine. But the flow of students towards medical profession is more and more important since their number in the first year has increased from 25,000 in 1969 to 35,000 in 1973.

One wonders what are the reasons which brought up this strong selection. Officially this limit is due to the number of medical students that can be reasonably accepted in hospitals during the last 3 years of the curriculum when these students undergo their clinical training. In fact it is considerably over the possibility of a qualified clinical teaching for each of these students. This decision was taken under the effect of contradictory pressures since demographical studies were unable to bring agreement between specialists in this field.

If this decision is maintained, according to the number of students engaged in the curriculum and if we admit that the 8,200 students in the second year will appear 7,000 as graduate, it can be evaluated that the number of practitioners will reach 150,000 in 1990 against 70,000 in 1973; medical density then will be of 260 for 100,000, which means more than one physician for 400 people. It seems difficult to appreciate the effect of this decision, which could be eventually revised in rise or in decrease by political decisions related to the economical situation, on the future of medical care in the country.

We shall make no comments on the number of students in pharmacy (which in 1973 is of 22,000 for 5 years of studies) and in dentistry: 8,250 for 4 years.

Whatsoever, it can be argued that from 1959 to 1969 in the University the proportion of students involved in medical care (Medicine, Pharmacy and Dentistry) has gone from 18 to 21% at the same moment when the total figure has practically tripled in 10 years, growing from 214,000 to 615,000.

On the other hand we have very precise figures on the number of people who are involved in schools directed by the Ministry of Health that is, in 1969, 37,128 pupils divided into:

nurses	25,644
masseurs	5,733
chiropodists	1,053
social helpers	4,698

These figures have practically not changed in 1973 but we shall discuss further the problems they bring up correlatively to what can be called 'the crisis of nurses.'

It is at present very difficult to evaluate the cost of teaching in medical and para-medical disciplines.

It should not exceed, in 1974, 2 billions francs divided into:

1,3 B for Universities
0,35 B for the Ministry of Health
0,25 B for National Health Insurance (very arbitrary estimation of expenses engaged by hospitals for teaching purposes)

The only reflection that can be made is that this cost seems to be very low when compared with the cost of sickness insurance which rises the same year to 64 B. It is certain that if economical situation would force a decrease in health expenses, this decrease could be compensated by a better education of medical staff and of patients. Large funds could be recovered from the cost of over-consumption of drugs and by reducing hospital stays. It is certain that such a decrease would be considered by the public like a social regression which explains why political power has up to now hesitated in solving this difficult problem of the growing cost of health.

Reflections about the French hospital-university complex and the system of medical education

The actual system of medical education is the result of two major events which have strongly influenced French politics. The first one has been, after a very serious reflection by a commission directed by Prof. Debré, the passing in 1958 of a Bill creating the Hospital-University Centres (C.H.U.) and giving a new status to professors in medicine. A second event is linked to the students' revolt in May 1968.

The Debré reform has given to French medical teaching and research a new development. It first has unified hospitals and university careers up to now divided and, by creating a full-time career with salaries doubling the former university wages, it has attached toward teaching and research the best students.

By increasing the number of teachers it has improved considerably the quality of medical education.

It failed on two important points:

1. It was unable, as was wanted at the beginning, to reduce the length of studies from 7 to 6 years.

2. It was unable to suppress the former system which limited to 40% by selection as 'externs' in hospitals, the number of students who got access to hospital responsibilities. On the other hand it was unable to impose the division of the huge faculty of medicine in Paris in spite of an excellent beginning in this way.

And finally the students reproached it to increase too much, in the first two years of the curriculum, basic sciences against clinical medicine. But the real reason of students' protestation was the demographical rush of the years 1967 and 1968 in medical schools which was going to bring a fast decline in the quality of teaching during the 1st two years of studies.

From May to October 1968, under the pressure of students, important reforms were hastily decided:

'Medicalisation' of the first year of studies

Hospital responsibilities for all the students from the 4th year of studies

The division in 10 medical Schools of the Faculty of Medicine in Paris

The application of the new law of 'orientation of the University' passed in November 1968 by the National Assembly has allowed the students to participate in the running of Universities and Units of Teaching and Research.

It is still too early to appreciate the results of these reforms.

Nevertheless we are authorised to say that this reform of 1968 would also have been without results if the limitation of the number of medical students had not been imposed, against the will of students' Unions, by the Ministry of Education. Since the number of students has been restricted to 8,200 admitted in the 2nd year, at the same time as the 26 faculties of medicine were transformed in 40 medical schools (10 in Paris, 4 in Lyon for example), the average number of students in each year is now of 200. This figure might appear high for U.S.A. and United Kingdom but it is a strong improvement compared with the former situation in France.

Between 1961 and 1971, the number of professors has risen from 1,920 to 2,862 and that of assistants and instructors from 3,800 to 6,147 but the number of students nearly tripled by that time. The situation, very difficult in 1971, should improve if the number of teachers continues to grow from 2 to 3% per year as it was the case these last 3 years, while the number of students will be decreasing slightly.

Reflections on the 'crisis' of nurses

The number of practising nurses was in 1972 of 123,000 divided in 63,000 in public hospitals, 40,000 in private hospitals and 20,000 in liberal practice. We must add to this number 38,200 nurses specialised in psychiatry.

Since the number of student nurses is more than 25,000 for 2 years

of studies and 28 months from 1974 it should be no problem in
recruiting. Unfortunately it seems that the average time of practice
of a nurse is no longer than between 5 and 8 years. These last 2 years
the problem has been acute, particularly in public hospitals, where
during holidays wards have had to be closed by shortage of nurses.

The main demands of the nurses concern low salaries, too hard
conditions of work and, may be also, lack of consideration from
doctors and patients. It is certain that a very strong effort still have
to be made on these 3 points. Possibility of part-time work has also
been proposed. The main problem is to decide if a strong improvement in all these conditions would necessarily increase the length
of the career for of nurses. So the problem for Health Authorities in
France is to know whether the main effort must be done on the
conditions of work or whether in any case it is necessary to largely
increase the number of students in the schools until we get balance.

Post-graduate retraining

A survey made upon doctors demonstrates that the average length
of work is around 50,4 hours per week. One must add 5 hours of
personal retraining. The medical unions have been involved, since
20 years, in collectively organising this retraining. Many groups of
permanent training have been constituted around the hospitals in
big and average towns. Teaching has been generally given freely
by the Professors of nearby universities. The frequency of these
meetings is of one evening per month. The cost of this organisation
is covered by the publicity budget of pharmaceutical firms. The
unions estimate that 15% of practitioners regularly attend these
meetings.

As far as specialists are concerned participation is more important
and the meetings generally take place at the University hospital.
Specialists have less obligations than practitioners and can easily
be free for a full day.

A very important bill has been passed in France in July 1971.
It constitutes in industry funds for permanent training which
represent in 1974 0,8% of salaries and could rise to 2% in the
future. The application of this bill in private firms brought very
quickly new organisms, public or private, for this new type of
training. Unfortunately the State, always late as far as its own
services are concerned, has not yet applied the bill to the public
function. Consequently no particular initiative has been taken for
the retraining of public hospital physicians.

A very strong discussion has established itself between medical
unions, public and powers to decide the financing of permanent

training of physicians in private practice and who will be in charge of the organisation. It could be a compulsory contribution for each physician or a financing brought about by the National Health Insurance which would be considered then as an employer. Medical unions have instituted a National Association which hopes to get the exclusivity of the permanent training. It is certain that this type of retraining should develop quickly.

It is estimated that the bulk of biological and medical knowledge is doubling every 10 years. Such an evolution should bring to reduce the length of medical studies at the beginning of the career and to organise permanent training. One speaks in the U.S.A. of a re-training with a control of knowledge which would be imposed every 6 years. Such a discipline would be excellent but when one knows the difficulty encountered in socialist countries, where the physicians are wage-earning, to impose permanent training of practitioners, one keeps sceptical of the possibility to generalise this training in the liberal system.

Medical Research

Such a study would not be complete if it did not concern the problem of relations between medical care and medical research. It can be said that progress in medical science is the main incentive to the growth of medical care. This has for France an important conse-quence: this growth is in fact essentially conditioned by discoveries made in the U.S.A. where expenses in medical research are 16 times higher than in France and 4 times higher when brought back to the number of inhabitants.

This large difference must not underestimate the effort made in France to develop medical research. Between 1955 and 1970 the annual growth-rate of INSERM has been of 38% against 10% for the National gross product and 14% for medical expenses. The number of scientists, a good expression of the growth is quantity, has risen, during the same period, of 19,2% per year. Indeed this growth has considerably diminished since 1970 when it is only of 5 to 6% per year but it remains definitely more important than the one of the whole of the French research.

The last global analysis of the effort for French research in the medical field, established in 1967, estimates public research expenses at 462 B francs and at 321 B the one of enterprises. The figures for 1974 should bring out a rise of 80 to 90% for the public expenses when compared with the 1957 figures.

These figures are far from being negligible even if they appear to be low when compared with medical consumption.

It clearly appears that political power has perfectly understood that even in an economy where growth-rate is decreasing the development of medical research must be maintained in order to reduce the expenses imposed by technical dependence towards foreign countries.

And finally it must be emphasised that in the fields where French medical research is good the quality of medical practice appears to be better than in other fields where no research is going on. For example an important effort of research has been done these last two years on the problems of perinatality and physiopathology of delivery where very few scientists were involved. It is evident that the development of several teams on these subjects is already improving the training of specialists in neo-natal paediatrics and in obstetrics.

Conclusion

Provision of medical care in France seems actually to satisfy both physicians and the population; the budget of the sickness insurance has increased in 1973 and 1974 by 15% against 10% for the National Gross Product. The main question is to know if such a growth will be tolerable in a context of economical crisis.

On the opposite it must be said that the situation is not so good as far as nurses, medical students and young physicians in public hospitals are concerned. When compared with the sickness insurance the budget of medical education appears to be relatively low and is far to follow the same annual progression. As a prudent suggestion in such a complex problem one may ask if some type of correlation between the budget of sickness insurance and the one of medical education could not improve the functioning of public hospitals which are involved, for most of them, in medical education.

Bibliography

Rapport sur l'organisation des études médicales—Mai 1970. La Documentation française (29-31 Quai Voltaire Paris 7).

Reflexions sur l'avenir du système de santé. La Documentation Française—Paris—1970.

Rösch, G—Economique Médicale. Flammarion—Paris—1973.

Santé et Sécurité Sociale Tableaux (edition 1972). La Documentation française—Paris—1973.

Chapter 12

SOME METHODOLOGICAL PROBLEMS OF INTERNATIONAL CO-OPERATION IN THE FIELD OF HEALTH

D. D. VENEDIKTOV
Ministry of Health of the USSR, Moscow, USSR

AT PRESENT many problems connected with the protection and promotion of human health, prophylaxis and treatment of diseases have become a matter of concern not only of physicians, scientists and other medical professional people, but also of general population, public figures and statesmen. These problems have acquired ever increasing social, political and even international significance and have occupied a prominent place in the activities of many governments and international organizations. This was caused by many reasons and, particularly, by the fact that after the 2nd World War mankind and the United Nations for the first time put a task of great importance—'the attainment of the highest level of health by all peoples' (WHO Constitution), considering it to be the universal benefit and direct responsibility of the States and Governments. Thus it implies that the most important social and international task is the attainment of the maximum level of health for each individual and for the whole of mankind at the present time and in future.

For all that the implication of 'health' as a complex and hardly measurable category was extended. Health is 'life, not restricted in its freedom' (K. Marx), 'a state of complete physical, mental and social well-being and not merely the absence of disease or infirmity' (WHO Constitution), 'equilibrium of the organism with the environment', it is a vital requirement and the basis for the harmonious development of the personality, indispensable condition for happiness, completeness of being and one of his inalienable rights; health is the greatest social and moral value, and also one of the basic goals of the socio-economic progress and one of its indispensable conditions, etc. Finally, health is one of the inalienable human rights secured by the international documents.

Various biological and social factors closely interlaced with each other (Figure I) influence the state of human health and the concepts of 'health' and 'health protection' are not only biological categories, but social as well and thus they should be considered and analysed within the framework of natural biological and social systems.

Recently in many countries and international organizations, at representative international congresses and more specialized meetings and also in general and special press, endless arguments and discussions have taken place on the past and future of the health protection and medical science, involving a wide range of problems: beginning with the role played by general practitioners or a hospital in a particular city and including the current and future problems of national and international health protection.

At the same time we can't help noticing that heated discussions on the problems of protection of the population's health very often come to nothing—they are lost in details and do not come to the point, do not provide a general idea of health protection, do not enable one to reveal the most common laws of the development of this activity. The difficulty becomes even greater due to the absence of the generally accepted international definition of the concept of 'health protection' (at least with the same degree of abstraction as 'health' was defined in the WHO Constitution). Internationally to describe measures directed to the protection and promotion of health of the individual and the society in English they use the words which in literal translation mean 'health services', while in French and Spanish—'public health', in Russian—'health protection', etc. It should be also taken into consideration that in many countries the words 'health protection' are supplemented with such vague epithets like 'communal', 'basic', 'primary', 'integrated', 'comprehensive', 'national', 'regional', etc., and as is stated in the Report compiled by the WHO Executive Board (1973) 'this list is far from being exhaustive and proves the complexity of the problem and the degree of erroneous translation resulting from confusion in terminology or expression and frequent substitution of one term by another'. Therefore specialists from various countries very often use diffused definitions for the concept of 'health protection' which had been given by K. E. Winslow, U. Farr, L. A. Shilley and many others many decades ago (E. L. Stebbins, 1965; F. Brockington, 1967; E. Amudsen et al., 1973).

Not underestimating the value of these definitions and the importance of the discussion on the specific problems and aspects of national and international health protection not infrequently we voiced at WHO sittings and in press the necessity of 'removal' of the above terminological 'blockages' so as to make the discussions of the adherents of various concepts in health protection essential rather than formal and to view the health services and systems in many countries from the most common and fundamental positions. In this respect the approach which was called the scientific systems approach to the society as a whole and to health protection and medical science was quite fruitful. The activity of separate medical institutions and different complexes of measures should be regarded in the light of historical evolution of the unified functional system of health protection for the population which the human society has been creating and implementing at different stages of its development and in any country. Basing on socio-systemic concepts we have proposed to define the concept of 'health protection' as 'a complex social dynamic functional system which is created and used by the society to implement the whole complex of social and medical measures aimed at the protection and continuous promotion of the health of every individual and the society as a whole, and, in particular, continuous development of medical research and accumulation of medical knowledge as the only possible basis of health protection; comprehensive individual and community measures of prophylaxis with special emphasis on the protection of health of the new generation and on environmental health, provision to the entire population for every possibility of timely diagnosis and high quality treatment of the diseases whenever they occur including rehabilitation and recurrence prophylaxis' (WHO A/26/20, p. 15).

The concept of socio-systemic and functional nature of health protection is based on the historical experience and the development of health protection in the USSR and other countries of the world, as well as on the theory of functional systems which has been fruitfully developed by P. K. Anokhin and is being developed nowadays by his followers, with regard to the higher nervous activity of man and systemic organization of biological functions. This concept has been frequently discussed at scientific conferences and in WHO and in a recently organized International Institute of Applied Systems Analysis in Laxenburg (Austria).

The Fifth WHO long-term programme for 1973–1977 reads: 'Health services occupy a very important place in the rapidly forming complex of political, economic, social, cultural, technical and psychological systems basing on the geophysical structure of the environment. Public health is represented in each of the above systems and, being an integral part of the general structure, effects it by its own dynamism' (WHA.24.58, p. 3). It also emphasizes that 'instead of being considered merely as a complex of solely medical measures, public health services are being recognized as an important component of socio-economic systems, combining all the economic, social, political, preventive, therapeutic and other measures which human society, in any country and at any stage in its development, is using to protect and constantly improve the health of every individual and of society as a whole'.

Each system is characterized, above all, by its own *goals* without which one cannot properly determine the 'boundaries' of the system. Claud Bernar used to say that 'medicine is a science, which aims at the protection of health and treatment of human diseases', thus emphasizing a very important thesis, well known from the ancient times, on the indissolubility of the combination of three basic elements of medicine: science, prevention and treatment.

But as the basic tasks of medicine of all times was the triad: to cognize the human organism and its possible disorders, prevent the diseases and cure them, whenever they occur, then even today all the diverse and numerous goals, tasks and functions of health services as a social dynamic system could ultimately be grouped in the following way:

a. Development of medical research and accumulation of medical knowledge as the only possible basis for all complex measures aimed at protection and promotion of human health;

b. Individual and community measures for prevention of diseases, with special emphasis on the protection of health of new generations and on environmental health as the main factor affecting human health;

c. Provision to the entire population of timely diagnosis of diseases and their adequate treatment whenever they occur and rehabilitation.

It should be noted here that the recognition of the insolubility of the above tasks not only in theory, but also in practice was very difficult before and is still uneasy now for the representatives of some countries, where these functions were 'traditionally' separated from each other and where health protection until recently was considered to be a 'private affair' of the patient and the sphere of the 'free' sale of services by practitioners.

However, life proves the impossibility of the solution of the problems of health protection and promotion, using private, personal or semi-social means and thus the far-sighted men of health services in all countries gradually come to the proper understanding of the interrelation and complex nature of the tasks, facing public health services (N. A. Semashko, 1963; M. Terris, 1972; M. G. Candau, 1971; W. Hobson, 1963; N. Goodman, F. Brockington, 1967; E. Aujauleau, 1970 and others).

Once again we should refer to the Fifth WHO long-term programme which says:

'Ultimately a conclusion can be drawn that there are three main tasks facing public health services: development of medical research and accumulation of medical and biological knowledge as the only possible basis for the complex measures aimed at health protection and promotion; comprehensive individual and community measures of prophylaxis, with special emphasis on the protection of health of the new generation and on environmental health; provision to the entire population of timely diagnosis of diseases and their adequate treatment whenever they occur and rehabilitation of the patients'.

It should be noted here, that of late, in many countries of the world much has been done with regards to systemic-structural analysis of health protection. Suffice it to refer you to the publications of WHO Headquarters, papers of the seminars of the Regional Office for Europe, technical discussions during the latest Sessions of the World Health Assembly, numerous monographs on the theory and practice of health protection in different countries, the attempts to make up 'models of health protection' for the states, cities and separate areas (H. Hillboe, 1971; J. Acton, R. Levin, 1971; F. Grunde and W. A. Reinke, 1973 and others), various publications on the economic analysis in the health field, etc. Thus the concept of systems approach may be considered to be sufficiently accepted and causes no principle objections.

Moreover it might be generally recognized that for the successful development and functioning of health care as a social system we have definite external and internal conditions. The external socio-economic and organizational conditions include, above all, reasonable approach to the protection of the health of the population as an important task of the community and the State and not as a private matter of a patient and a physician; high level of economic and technological development as the only basis for the effective health protection of the population and, finally, training of qualified medical cadres of various categories and continuous growth of the educational, cultural and sanitary level of the entire population.

The following principles could be referred to the number of internal conditions or principles of the formation of the effective health care system : the expediency of its state unique and planned nature, its scientific basis, preventive trends, coverage with medical care of the entire population, indissoluble connections with the population, thus enjoying its support and faith, etc.

WHO World Health Assembly in its resolution 23.61 recommends these principles to all Member-States for planning and formation of national health protection systems and services, with regards to the specific national, historical, socio-economic and other conditions, as 'the most effective and proved in practice by a number of countries'. Therefore we shall not discuss these conditions at length but we shall show you the diagram reflecting the above conditions in brief (Figure 3).

While analysing the systems and health services in different countries, one should remember that they function under rapidly changing conditions, and the most important shifts that take place in the external situation and under internal conditions of health systems are specific for this or that country, and at the same time, they have much in common, characteristic of a number of countries and regions or for all countries of the world. We shall illustrate this thesis by several external and internal shifts which affect essentially the activities of health bodies in many countries, their strategy and tactics (Figure 4).

Among the most important 'external' shifts are the following:

a. Economic shifts (industrial and agricultural). Complication of economic relations. Industrialization. Acceleration of communication and transportation. Scientific-technological revolution. Aggravation of social and class contradictions.

b. Urbanization and growth of the urban population. Increase of the educational level. Increase of mass information. Psychological stress, caused by an increased tempo of life.

c. Population growth. Involvement of women into labour process. Accelerated development of children and minors. Relative 'ageing' of the population.

d. Environmental pollution (water, soil, air). Ecological shifts.

e. Changes in the state of health, morbidity and mortality patterns of the population. Shifts in the nutritional statute and 'chemicalization' of the population. Harmful habits.

The 'internal' shifts are the following:

a. Progress in medico-biological science, prerevolutionary state of a number of branches of science. Increase of the complexity and expenditures on research.

b. Success, attained in the control of epidemic and communicable diseases, and changes in the conditions of their global spread. Lack of the current and preventive sanitary control.

c. Increase of the cost of medical care. Elaboration of the new methods of treatment of terminal and severe states, improvement of equipment and enlargement of medical establishments.

d. Shortage (in many countries) of qualified medical personnel, research and auxiliary cadres and a slow tempo of their training. Development of 'team methods' in rendering medical care. Negative effect of the 'brain drain' from developing countries to highly developed ones.

e. Uneven coverage with medical care of urban and rural population and also (in many countries) of various strata and groups of population. The growing necessity to equalize the volume and the quality of curatice-preventive care.

The complexity of health systems is aggravated by the fact that a whole number of theoretical and practical problems of medicine which have earlier been of interest only for a limited number of specialists and Governments of some countries, nowadays outgrew national borders and turned out to be international and global health problems which can be solved by the united efforts of governments of many countries and international organizations.

Among these problems are, specifically, the following (Figure 5):

a. Accelerated development and international co-operation of medico-biological research aiming at fundamental solution of the essential theoretical and practical problems of medicine;

b. Struggle against the dangerous *epidemic diseases* (smallpox, plague, cholera, yellow fever, etc.), making use of global surveillance of epidemiological processes and with due regard for the peculiarities of the spread of epidemics in the age of high-speed communication and transport.

c. The study and elaboration of preventive and curative methods against non-epidemic *major diseases*: cardio-vascular disorders, cancer, congenital disorders, viral infections, etc.

d. Medical aspects of protection and improvement of the environment including the establishment of international standards for maximum permissible concentrations of various substances in the air, water and soil; protection of the world ocean and the atmosphere.

e. Guarantee of the *effective control over the quality, safety, efficacy and side-effects of drugs* and steps directed against voluntary and involuntary abuse of various medicines in connection with the broad development of the pharmaceutical and chemical industries and of international trade.

f. Assistance to the developing countries in the organization and development of the effective national systems and services of public health and in training of national medical cadres.

g. Socio-hygienic study of the *population dynamics* and changes *in the structure*, birth-rate, death-rate and morbidity to elaborate a new health strategy. This is closely linked with the problem of ensuring sufficient and balanced nutrition of the population and with the struggle against illnesses connected with *malnutrition and starvation*, as well as with the general questions of the future dynamics of the population growth in view of both positive and negative consequences of the scientific-technological progress for health of the mankind.

The scope of the above medico-social problems make international co-operation in the health field and medicine necessary practically for all countries of the world.

For the past decades international co-operation in the health field has become extremely diverse in its forms, scale methods and forces, so that there is every ground to speak of the 'international health' as the most important field of activities for health services in all countries of the world, we may also speak of the international legal regulation or even of the already formed or being formed international, functional social system, aimed at exchange of experience and information in the health field between different countries and ultimate solution of the objective international and global medico-social problems.

The development of the above collaboration requires great efforts and, in particular, mutual understanding between different countries (including unique and similar terminology), mutual compatibility between certain elements of the national health systems and services; and in future—the elaboration of new international methodology to assist the solution of the most pressing problems. It is in this field that the most important role of WHO and other international, inter-governmental and non-governmental organizations is played. It should also be taken into consideration that a long time will pass since the moment of recognition of the health services as a functional system and determination of the basic principles of its optimal activity and the moment of its practical, implementation; this could be compared with the moment of designing a house and the moment it has been erected. This distance should be covered in no time, using the experience of different countries and the available methodology.

One of the first steps, in our opinion, may be the formation of the generalized model of health services as a functional system, its logical, mathematical and organizational description.

From this point of view there might be suggested the health management model for a definite administrative-territorial unit (State, Republic, City, etc.). Each administrative territory has a more or less branched network of health bodies and health establishments of different degree of centralization, including (Figure 6) *research institutions* (Medical Schools, Laboratories, groups, etc.); Higher and Secondary *medical establishments*; *Sanitary-anti-epidemic establishments*; which provide preventive and everyday control and carry out anti-epidemic measures; *curative-prophylactic* in- and out-patient establishments, which provide various types of medical care to the local population and visitors; pharmaceutical, technical, supply, repair and other services and organizations.

Finally, each territory has *one or several Health Bodies* which combine (or should combine) territorial subordination to the local governmental bodies with the subordination to the higher standing body.

At the same time, all medical establishments, located at the given territory, independent of their subordination, should not only provide medical care to the population residing in the given location, but also meet the requirements of the whole network of the national health system and function in accordance with the principles and standards of the above system. Each medical establishment may and should (by its functions or results) come into the composition of various systems' hierarchies: medical science, education, sanitary epidemiological services, preventive and therapeutic establishments, health management services etc. Proper combination of all functions of the above establishments which meet the requirements of each geographical location of the country will, in all probability, be optimal for the solution of the basic tasks, facing health services.

The experience of many years standing showed that co-ordination and planning of research and training of medical personnel are the vital functions and are of centralized nature. Preventive and anti-epidemic services should be brought as close as possible to the population and be able for immediate mobilization and centralization in case of need at the national and international level. Medical care to the population should be built on the basis of echelonment or staged nature of diagnostic and curative services, providing urgent medical care not only to the local population, but also to a definite contingent of migrating population. As it has already been said, health management should by all means combine subordination to local authorities and administrative bodies to provide for active participation of the community and governmental bodies in the implementation of necessary medical measures with direct subordination to the higher standing health bodies to result in unique actions within the framework of the whole health system all over the territory of the given country.

No doubt the modelling is a very complicated affair and the suggested model is an abstract and conventional one. However, this model is sufficiently universal and could be easily applied in any country. In the course of discussions in WHO we emphasized the necessity of adopting the above model in the health field, like one can can accept in principle the model of the automobile, aircraft or other technological system. This model should foresee all the basic units and their interrelation, without which the system will fail to function.

The proposed generalized model of the health system may be taken as a basis for the elaboration of more detailed health models, increasing in their complexity—regarding both inferior bodies (a specific medical establishment) and superior bodies (the whole network of health services). However, it has its disadvantages: it is a static and non-operative one, it does not contain general efficacy criteria and those of certain functions and organizations, it does not define the concept of optimal centralization and decentralization of the system, etc.

Further elaboration and detailing of the model requires, therefore, a more thorough *analysis of each of the basic functions of health services*, with due regard for different terminology and units of measurement (if any) of each function including such as 'requirements', 'demands', 'maximum', minimum' and 'optimum' in meeting each of these requirements; availability of additional functions and their interrelation with the basic functions, etc. Particular attention should be paid to the efficacy criteria of the health services management, taking into consideration the structural differences of health bodies and establishments in different countries, trying to select such a range of countries which would have transitional phases, i.e. which would have definite differences and some similar features.

Of interest in this respect are the results of the WHO/Regional Office for Europe Working Group (Stockholm, June 1972) on the problems of health planning within the framework of national development. This Group divided all countries of Europe into three basic groups: the first group consists of Bulgaria, Hungary, Poland, Rumania, USSR, Czechoslovakia and, partially, Yugoslavia, with centralized systems of health services, where 'the plans of health development are the integral part of the general state plans of the socio-economic development'. The second group includes Belgium, Netherlands, Great Britain, Turkey, France, Sweden and other countries, characterized by 'sufficiently wide processes of planning', where the obtained results 'as basic indications of the general trends, rather than the means of elaboration of the detailed plan to be approved by the Government'. The third group consists of Austria, Italy and Spain, where 'the elements of planning of health services exist, but on a much smaller scale', compared with the other two groups.

Naturally, comparison of the health services and functions in different countries of the world should be carried out not in statics, but with due regard for the historical evolution of each function and every type of establishment in various countries and contemporary legal acts and rulings. This will enable one to reveal the similarity of health bodies and institutions, which have a different name, structure, subordination, etc. in different countries.

A question of information facilities of the health services and systems of today and rational means and ways of utilization of electronic computers in the health field deserves great attention. At present health systems in many countries are characterized by large volumes and flows of extremely diverse data, and not infrequently these data are found to be very complicated and interlaced with each other, and with the abundance of secondary data one very often fails to find the necessary information for the solution of the pressing problems. Complete coverage of medical, epidemiological, statistical and other information is usually accompanied by its substantial losses at various stages of processing and by the information 'noise', the selective registration of data, however, does not always yield sufficiently reliable indices and conclusions.

For many years health bodies and establishments in many countries of the world cherished great hopes for accelerated processing of the traditional statistical and other data by means of computers, and they did achieve some success.

It is known that in a number of countries, such as USA, Great Britain, France, Japan, Sweden, USSR, GDR, Bulgaria, Poland and others, electronic computers are widely used for the solution of health problems, mainly by means of local information-computing systems, covering the activities of certain medical establishments or kinds of functions, aiming at further increase and integration of the existing local systems into regional and even national computer centres in specific branches of health services. In some cases highly capacious Computer Centres are set up, which serve more than one hospital or medical establishment. Books, articles, scientific conferences and meetings, including those held by WHO, are dedicated to the problem of utilization of computers and systems technology in the health field. Such conferences and symposia took place, for instance, in Kiel (September, 1967), Bucharest (September, 1969), Copenhagen (February, 1970), Bratislava (February, 1970), Geneva (September, 1971), Luxemburg (July, 1972), Washington (April, 1973), etc.

At present there are two basic trends for computer utilization in medicine: First—for the analysis and management of biological systems (modelling of biological systems, automation of clinical and laboratory tests, automated diagnosis, long-term follow-up of patients and prognostication of the course of the disease); second—for the management of various elements and components of the health system as a social system (processing of statistical data and primary sources of medical information, hospital management, scientific-medical information, economic analysis and health prognosis, etc.) (Figure 7).

Alongside with this, even today, there is a confusion in the methods of computer utilization in the health field, incompatibility of the initial and final data, incompatibility of the systems or computer processing of medical information etc. Therefore we insistently raise the question of elaboration of unified principles of medical information processing in the health systems of different countries to facilitate mutual exchange of information and co-operation. This is a great and noble task, facing WHO and IIASA.

We should also take into account various approaches to the above problem. In the USSR the attempts are made to create a unified Branch Automated System of Management (BASM) of the health services for the whole country (BASM—'Health'). This is a complex system based on the interrelated subsystems at the level of Union, Republic, oblast or city and institution or hospital (Figure 8).

The development of BASM should lead to management improvement at every level to render better medical and preventive care for adults and children in urban and rural areas including specialized types of medical care; it should lead to prevention and eradication of epidemics, development of the sanitary-epidemiological service; perfection of the drug supply system and management of pharmaceutical industry; perfection of training of medical personnel, distribution and utilization of medical and pharmaceutical staff of the health service; perfection of the network planning and of current activities of medical institutions; optimization of financing of health and research institutions by means of proper finance control and accounting; perfection of the analysis of medico-statistical data, better use of the scientific medical and medico-technical information (Figure 9).

Electronic computers are necessary for the creation of the international system of medical and medico-technical information, the system of the global sanitary-epidemiological surveillance, co-ordination of medical research and also for the creation of the control system over the quality and efficacy of pharmaceutical preparations in the international trade and the study of side-effects of medicinal preparations etc.

The problems of health economy also deserve serious investigation and systemic analysis; they are called to supply the answers to the two main questions: first, what is the optimal amount of means and efforts that the mankind should spend to meet the requirements of the health service, and, second, how should we spend the available resources in a highly rational way and with maximum efficacy. Much information was published in press of late on the economy analysis of the activities of certain medical establishments and health service with the comparison of the obtained economic effect and undertaken efforts, etc. The problem of applicability of direct economic criteria for the assessment of the activity of health services and what economic aspects of health services should be developed and to what extent, is debated heatedly. In our opinion, of primary importance are the theoretical aspects of the health economy problem, as their direct application 'in practice' (the choice of therapeutic methods, depending on their costs, economic justification of the therapy of the aged and hopelessly sick, etc.) is rather dangerous. We agree with those economists who state that even economy as such cannot be analysed from purely economic positions. This is also true of health service, where the value of life and health of a human being cannot be directly expressed in monetary units. Such an 'economy' may seriously complicate the health system development and undermine the prestige of the medical profession people, although it is quite evident that at the national level we should register all the available resources and plan them in the most effective way. We advocate a careful and serious approach to the problems of health economy and agree with S. M. Danyushevsky (1967), V. V. Golovteev (1972) and others, who, when speaking of the health system's contribution to the countries' economy, emphasize that up till now nobody could differentiate numerous socio-economic and biological factors affecting the health of the population and purely medical ones (therapeutic, preventive, sanitary-epidemiological, etc.). Therefore despite the great number of papers on the analysis of expenditures on public health and their repayment, they all are of relative value.

An important task is elaboration of the methods for long-term planning and health prognosis with due regard for the objective trends and prospects of the community development and the systems of national and international health protection. At present in many countries scientists are trying to prognosticate the development of economy, science and technology with the coverage of all spheres of the social community life up to 1980, 1990 and 2000. Similar work is carried out in the health field on the national and international levels, but the prognoses could not be compared or analysed from the methodological point of view, with due account of all complex health interrelations and health subsystems within all the spheres of community life. We believe this to be a direct task of WHO and IIASA. It seems reasonable to prognosticate in the health field along three fundamental lines :

a. Prognoses of the development of medico-biological science;
b. Prognoses of the conditions of community life;
c. Prognoses of the future development of national and international health systems.

Further, we shall only concentrate of the prognostication and development of medico-biological science, including possible scientific discoveries and their perspective application in practical health field. One should not only forsee all the 'breakthroughs' and great discoveries in the coming years of the universal scientific-technological revolution, but also get them tied up with the research carried out all over the world and the perspectives for the international scientific co-operation.

Nowadays medicine and biology investigate practically all the existing and possible points of contact of a human being with the environment. Here, on the one hand, the united 'scientific front' of medicine and biology has already been formed, while, on the other hand, this 'front' has split into innumerable specialized trends, sectors and areas. The advancement of the scientific 'front', when a human being continuously discloses one secret of a nature after another, is irregular.

The first aspect of the irregularity in the development of science is the *acceleration* of the tempo of the development of medicine and biology in the course of scientific-technological revolution, compared with other branches of natural science, and it is quite probable that immediately after the remarkable discoveries and achievements of physics, chemistry and energetics, it is biology and medicine that may take the first place among other sciences (V. D. Timakov, 1972; N. P. Dubinin, 1972; V. A. Engelgart, 1970; P. K. Anokhin, 1970; B. M. Kedrov, J. Tilling-Smith, Mattis, D. King-Hilley, 1969; G. Taylor, 1968 and others).

The XXV World Health Assembly, which took place in May, 1972 also stressed in its resolution WHA 25.60 that 'in the course of the accelerated scientific-technological progress, science turns out into the productive force of the community and that we have every ground to believe that, in nearest future, all significant discoveries in the field of biology and medicine, may have essential social and economic importance'.

The second aspect of irregularity of the development of medicine and biology is the unequal tempo of the development of certain trends of this very complicated scientific complex. While certain trends develop rather quietly, the other branches of biology and medicine are found to have high concentration of scientific means, and unexpected events and seemingly paradoxical conclusions, in our opinion, make us expect possible 'pre-breakthrough', 'pre-thunder' or even 'pre-revolutionary' state of the above scientific trends. The irregularity of the development results from the complexity of interrelations and interinfluences of various medico-biological scientific disciplines on each other and on other adjacent branches of natural science.

The comparison of the whole number of governmental and inter-national scientific-planned documents with regards to medicine and biology, proves that at present, in the majority of countries the basic efforts of scientists and research medico-biological institutions are concentrated to a great extent at some very important trends and problems and at definite methodological levels of their study (Figure 10). In terms of problems the most important are those 'diseases of the age' as cardio-vascular disorders, cancer and other malignant tumors, infectious, viral and bacterial diseases, genetic defects and congenital diseases, the dependency of the state of health of a human being on the environmental factors and a number of others.

All the above problems are being developed simultaneously at different methodological levels, each of them, in itself, presents a very important stage of analysis and cognition of the biological processes, as well as it represents an independent field of knowledge and a branch of science. The most important level is that of molecular biology and cellular genetics, organization of intact and functional biological systems, general and particular immunology, the study of the individual development of the human organism, the study of psychology and behavioral sciences, and, finally, socio-hygienic aspects of each medical problem and the problems of scientific management of health and of the science itself.

The problem and methodological approach in contemporary biology and medicine are absolutely natural, necessary and are closely inter-connected with each other. Moreover, the most important discoveries and 'breakthroughs' are prognosed basically at these points of contact or crosspoints, and not only every problem could be successfully solved on the basis of multilateral methodological approach, but at the same time every scientific methodological level may greatly contribute to the study of various problems.

The third aspect of irregularity in the advancement of the medico-biological scientific front is the difference in the degree of the development of theoretical and applied research *in different countries*, which could be associated with their different economic and scientific-technological potential, and also with the attention, paid by the Governments of the respective countries to medical science and health services.

Alongside with this, it becomes more evident that even the very highly developed countries are not able to successfully develop the necessary and perspective medico-biological, fundamental and applied research with their own efforts.

This is not only a question of huge expenses, but, above all, a question of the complexity of problems facing the science and requiring united efforts of not only individual scientists and teams of scientists, but many countries as well.

However, the development of genuine international co-operation in the medical and biological field is a complicated matter, and, at present, this co-operation is impeded by at least three 'barriers'—information, methodological and socio-ethic ones. It is quite evident that this comparison is purely conventional, it would be more proper to speak of the complex of problems connected with the *scientific-information* provision of science, *methodology* of international co-operation and realization of the ever increasing *social responsibility* of science and scientists.

Contrary to other branches of science (for instance, nuclear physics or exploration of space) which simultaneously developed in many countries of the world, which enabled to make up the unique terminology and similar methodological approaches, and in contrast to technology, which developed from simplified machines to more complicated ones, medicine proceeded for ages from primitive scientific empirism, with a human being and his diseases as the only object of investigation, the complexity of which greatly exceeds the 'resolution' of all past and contemporary methods of investigation which are developed in different countries in their own way. Medicine even nowadays uses a great number of empiric methods of therapy, which but gradually receive scientific explanation.

This resulted in a situation, too well known to the medical profession people when often one and the same terms designate in different countries various forms of diseases or phases of their progressing (according to WHO, contemporary medicine uses more than 20,000 terms, the majority of which are obsolete both in essence and form). On the other hand, it is often the case that practically similar pathological processes and diseases are described with different terms.

Finally, the scientific-technological revolution of today disclosed the increased role of science as a social institution and an important factor of community development, as well as the difficulties and contradictions, adherent to this institution. This led to the increase of responsibility of scientists, heated discussions on the role and place of science in the community life, on mutual connections and impact of the scientific-technological and social progress, etc.

This finds its direct reflection in medical science, which has always been not only theoretical, but a practical applied discipline. And since the social conditions in every country are of paramount importance, it is not accidental, then, that at present there is a great gap between *what can already be done* by science today for protection and promotion of human health and *what is being done* in practice for the population of many countries of the world, both developing and highly developed ones, and this fact is of ever increasing social significance.

Another aspect of the socio-ethic barrier is the problem of 'free' theoretical investigations in contrast to applied investigations, and of late great interest was aroused by the problem of permissible limits of experiments, carried out on a human being in the process of medico-biological studies. A number of Declarations and Codes of medical ethics are dedicated to this problem (Nurnberg Code, Helsinki Declaration, Sydney Declaration, etc.). This problem was also covered by a number of international symposia and conferences (SIOMS symposia in 1972 and 1973, 'CIBA' symposium in 1971 and many others). ECOSOS, UN, UNESCO and WHO deal with the problem of the 'rights of a human being in the process of medico-biological investigations' (within the framework of WHO there is a Special Secretariat on Moral and Ethic Aspects of ALL Scientific Investigations, which are carried out under the auspices of WHO). However, the problem remains acute, moreover, that of late scientists require the revision of the Code on medical ethics, which reads on the prolongation of life for grave and chronic cases and euthanasia for hopeless patients. And, finally, serious is the problem of the further perspectives and remote consequences of medico-biological discoveries (manipulations with the genetic code, functions of the human brain, etc.), and social responsibility of science. Some scientists voice pessimistic ideas and nihilism with regards to future; they consider the social problems of the utilization of the future achievements of medicine and biology as extremely acute, insoluble, extremely dangerous and even ominous (G. Taylor, P. Harper, S. F. Powell, 1969; O. Toffler and others) and propose to cease a number of medico-biological investigations or decree 'the moratorium' (J. Pickering, 1966; M. Burnett, 1971 and others). We do not share this pessimism, but may emphasize once again the importance of the pronounced assumption, which was also voiced by the World Health Assembly, that 'the achievements of medicine and biology, the most humane of all sciences, should be used only for the benefit and never to destroy mankind'.

Alongside with this, the international co-operation in the health field is not only a desirable condition of its further development, but also a real and irreversible fact of contemporary life. Therefore, we do not only mean a mere recognition of this fact, but an increase of the international scientific collaboration, development of its methodology, based on the universal interest in the results of medico-biological investigations and voluntary participation of all countries, inadmissibility of external interference, pressure or dictate executed on national scientific establishments.

We consider that in future WHO will play a greater role in the development of scientific medicine, and in the WHA resolution 25.60 'On the role of WHO in the development and co-ordination of medico-biological research' which was adopted according to the proposal, advanced by the USSR, USA, Great Britain, France, Poland, Czechoslovakia, Hungary, Bulgaria and other countries it is stated that WHO will implement:

'1. detection and promotion of the development of those fields of medico-biological science, which seem to be most promising, from the point of view of future results; 2. development and perfection of the methods and possibilities of international co-operation in the field of medico-biological science, standardization of scientific methods of investigations, standardization of nomenclature and terminology, whenever possible, to provide the comparability of results; 3. co-ordination of research efforts in the countries, which will display readiness to provide the necessary facilities and staff for the joint work on the problems of primary importance; 4. accumulation and presentation of information to the Member-States with regards to the most rational ways of practical utilization of the research achievements in health programmes; 5. provision of methodological training to research fellows, especially young ones, who wish to participate in medico-biological research, and also in the assessment of the above research and results'.

It is quite evident that the efforts of WHO and other international organizations should be aimed, in the first head, at those research-medical problems, that present great interest and significance for all the countries, and should be supported by the specific (in contrast to national) methodology of co-ordination of national efforts.

It seems to us that the basic principles of the methodology of international research programmes should be the establishment of the priority in medico-biological problems, which require international co-ordination; registration and analysis of ideas and prognoses for the solution of the above problems compilation of the complex plans for the co-ordinated study and development of these problems, having in mind maximum utilization of the national efforts of the Member-States and implementation with international efforts of the most important tasks and research; provision of the systematic registration and assessment of the achieved results on the international programmes and introduction of the corresponding corrections into the future plans. All this may make is possible to execute such international research-medical co-operation, which will be aimed not only at the study, but, ultimately, at the solution of the most important medico-biological and international socio-hygienic problems, which are of great interest for all the countries of the world.

Here, the International Institute of Applied Systems Analysis (IIASA) might greatly contribute, jointly with WHO, to the solution of a whole number of methodological problems from the systems and analytical points of view. It seems to us, that the most interesting problems in this regards are—the analysis of the contemporary research-medical potential, comparison of prognoses of the development of medico-biological science, the study of scientific information systems and elaboration of the information, systemic and mathematical provision of research programmes.

The first programme of this kind may be the Programme of international Co-operation in the field of oncology, which is being developed in accordance with the WHO resolution 26.61 'under the auspices of WHO, IACR, IOU and other international bodies in correspondence with their Rules and Regulations.

The problems of the elaboration of the international oncological programme have been widely discussed at the 27th World Health Assembly in May 1974 in Geneva, and its practical implementation has already started. The success or failure of the programme largely depend not only on the wish of the scientists of many WHO Member-States to join their efforts in practical solution of this most acute problem of medicine of today, but also whether effective and reliable methodology of this international co-operation will be elaborated. Should this be the case, the International oncological programme will become a prototype of other international medical scientific programmes, carried out on a large scale.

We do hope that will be the case.

References

Acton, J., Levine, R. *State health manpower planning: a policy overview.* The Rand Corporation, California, 1971.

Amundsen, E. *The problem of integrating health planning with socio-economic planning.* In: Interrelationships between health programmes and socio-economic development. Public Health Papers, 1973, 49, 27–32.

Aujaleu, E. *Prospective studies and future action in the public health field.* CESP, 1970.

Brockington, F. *World Health.* London, J. & A. Churchill Ltd., 1967.

Brunet-Jailly, J. *Essai sur l'économie général de la santé.* Paris, Cujas, 1971.

Candau, M. G. *The challenge of medical research.* WHO Chronicle, 1972, 26, 8, 335–338.

Goodman, N. M. *International health organizations and their work.* Edinburgh and London, Churchill Livingstone, 1971.

Grundy, F. & Reinke, W. A. *Health practice research and formalized managerial methods.* Public Health Papers, 51, WHO, Geneva, 1973.

Hilleboe, H. E. *Preventing future shock: health developments in the 1960's and imperatives for the 1970's* (The 11th Bronfman lecture.) A.J.P.H., 1972, Feb., 136–151.

Hobson, W. *World health and history.* Bristol, John Wright & Sons Ltd., 1963.

Scheele, L. A. *Public Health 1852–1952.* Journal of the Mount Sinai Hospital, Symposium on Medicine and Society. Baltimore, 1953, 764–789.

Taylor, G. R. *The biological time-bomb.* Thames & Hudson, London, 1968.

Tilling-Smith, G. *Health economics and cost-benefit analysis.* In: Health Planning and Organization of Medical Care. WHO, Copenhagen, 1972, 34–45.

Terris, M. *The need for a national health program.* Bull. N.Y. Acad. Med., 1972, 48, 1, 24–31.

Winslow, C. E. A. *Evolution of Public Health.* Oxford, 1923.

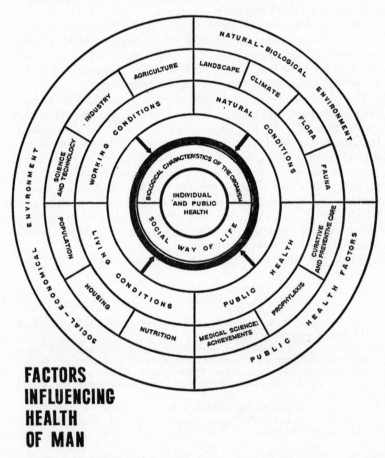

FACTORS INFLUENCING HEALTH OF MAN

Fig. 1.

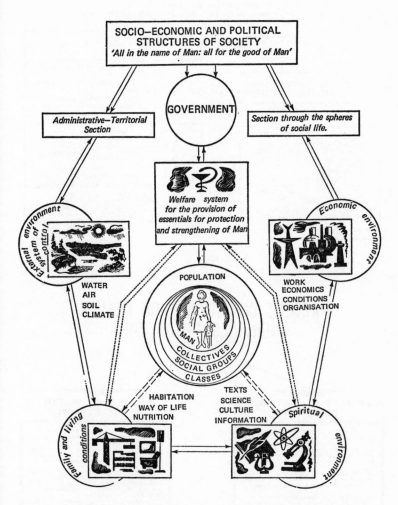

Fig. 2. The Place of the Welfare System in Society and its Links with Public Life

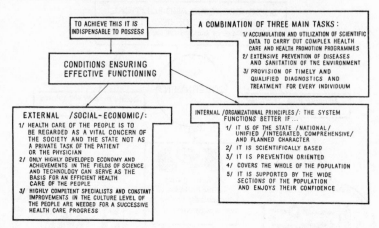

OBJECTIVES AND CONDITIONS OF THE HEALTH DEVELOPMENT
/AS A COMPLEX PUBLIC DYNAMIC SYSTEM /

OBJECTIVE OF THE SYSTEM EXISTENCE:
HEALTH CARE AND UNCEASING HEALTH PROMOTION FOR EVERY INDIVIDUAL AND THE SOCIETY AS A WHOLE

TO ACHIEVE THIS IT IS INDISPENSABLE TO POSSESS

A COMBINATION OF THREE MAIN TASKS:
1/ ACCUMULATION AND UTILIZATION OF SCIENTIFIC DATA TO CARRY OUT COMPLEX HEALTH CARE AND HEALTH PROMOTION PROGRAMMES
2/ EXTENSIVE PREVENTION OF DISEASES AND SANITATION OF THE ENVIRONMENT
3/ PROVISION OF TIMELY AND QUALIFIED DIAGNOSTICS AND TREATMENT FOR EVERY INDIVIDUUM

CONDITIONS ENSURING EFFECTIVE FUNCTIONING

EXTERNAL /SOCIAL-ECONOMIC/:
1/ HEALTH CARE OF THE PEOPLE IS TO BE REGARDED AS A VITAL CONCERN OF THE SOCIETY AND THE STATE NOT AS A PRIVATE TASK OF THE PATIENT OR THE PHYSICIAN
2/ ONLY HIGHLY DEVELOPED ECONOMY AND ACHIEVEMENTS IN THE FIELDS OF SCIENCE AND TECHNOLOGY CAN SERVE AS THE BASIS FOR AN EFFICIENT HEALTH CARE OF THE PEOPLE
3/ HIGHLY COMPETENT SPECIALISTS AND CONSTANT IMPROVEMENTS IN THE CULTURE LEVEL OF THE PEOPLE ARE NEEDED FOR A SUCCESSIVE HEALTH CARE PROGRESS

INTERNAL /ORGANIZATIONAL PRINCIPLES/: THE SYSTEM FUNCTIONS BETTER IF...
1/ IT IS OF THE STATE /NATIONAL/ UNIFIED /INTEGRATED, COMPREHENSIVE/ AND PLANNED CHARACTER
2/ IT IS SCIENTIFICALLY BASED
3/ IT IS PREVENTION ORIENTED
4/ COVERS WHOLE OF THE POPULATION
5/ IT IS SUPPORTED BY THE WIDE SECTIONS OF THE POPULATION AND ENJOYS THEIR CONFIDENCE

Fig. 3.

PRESENT CONDITIONS FOR HEALTH SERVICES OPERATION

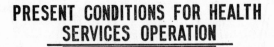

A. CHANCES IN «EXTERNAL» CONDITIONS

a) PROGRESS IN INDUSTRY AND AGRICULTURE. COMPLICATION OF THE ECONOMIC CONTACTS. INDUSTRIALIZATION. GROWTH OF COMMUNICATION AND TRANSPORT. SCIENTIFIC TECHNOLOGICAL REVOLUTION. INTENSIFICATION OF SOCIAL AND CLASS CONTRADICTIONS.

b) URBANIZATION. EDUCATION GROWTH. INTENSIFICATION OF MASS INFORMATION. PSYCHOLOGICAL STRESS AND MODERN SPEED OF LIFE.

c) POPULATION GROWTH. INTRODUCTION OF WOMEN INTO SOCIAL LABOUR. ACCELERATION. RELATIVE «AGEING» OF THE POPULATION.

D) ENVIRONMENTAL POLLUTION (OF WATER, SOIL, AIR), ECOLOGICAL CHANGES.

e) VARIATIONS IN HEALTH STATUS, IN THE MORBIDITY AND MORTALITY STRUCTURES. CHANGES IN DIET AND «CHEMIZATION» OF THE POPULATION. HARMFUL HABITS

B. INTERNAL SHIFTS IN THE SYSTEMS:

a) IMPETUOUS GROWTH OF BIOMEDICAL SCIENCES. INCREASE OF THE SCIENCE COMPLEXITY AND EXPENDITURES.

b) CONTROL OF EPIDEMICS IN THE CHANGING CONDITIONS OF THEIR GLOBAL PREVALENCE. INSUFFICIENCY OF CURRENT AND PREVENTIVE HEALTH INSPECTION.

c) INCREASE OF MEDICAL CARE COSTS. NEW METHODS OF TREATING TERMINAL AND GRAVE CONDITIONS. GROWTH OF TECHNICAL EQUIPMENT AND ENLARGEMENT OF MEDICAL AND HEALTH ESTABLISHMENTS.

d) SHORTAGE (IN MANY COUNTRIES) OF QUALIFIED MEDICAL, SCIENTIFIC AND AUXILIARY MANPOWER AND A SLOW RATE OF THEIR PREPARATION. DEVELOPMENT OF «TEAM WORK» METHODS IN HEALTH CARE. NEGATIVE EFFECTS OF «BRAIN DRAIN»

e) UNEVEN HEALTH SERVICES COVERAGE OF URBAN AND RURAL POPULATION AND (IN MANY COUNTRIES) OF DIFFERENT SOCIAL STRATA AND POPULATION GROUPS. A NEED TO EQUALIZE AN EXTEND AND QUALITY OF CURATIVE-REVENTIVE CARE

Fig. 4.

INTERNATIONAL /GLOBAL/ HEALTH PROBLEMS

1. INTERNATIONAL COORDINATION OF BIOMEDICAL RESEARCH

2. EPIDEMICS CONTROL AND GLOBAL EPIDEMIOLOGICAL SURVEY

3. RESEARCH, PREVENTION AND CONTROL OF CARDIOVASCULAR, TUMOUR AND OTHER MAJOR DISEASES

4. ENVIRONMENTAL HEALTH AND PROTECTION OF BIOSPHERE

5. CONTROL OVER THE QUALITY, EFFECTIVENESS AND SIDE EFFECTS OF DRUGS

6. ASSISTANCE TO NATIONAL HEALTH SERVICES AND HEALTH MANPOWER TRAINING IN THE DEVELOPING COUNTRIES

7. POPULATION DYNAMICS AND NUTRITION

Fig. 5.

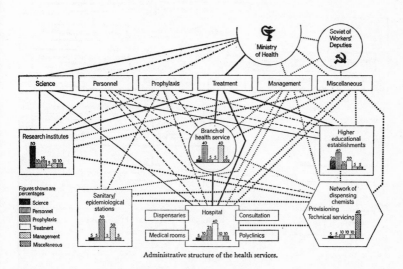

Administrative structure of the health services.

Fig. 6.

MAIN DIRECTIONS
IN THE COMPUTER APPLICATION IN MEDICINE

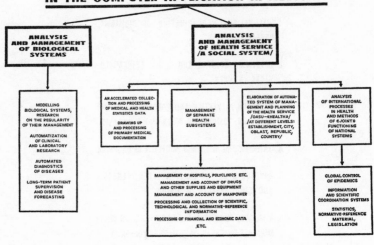

Fig. 7.

AUTOMATED SYSTEM OF THE MANAGEMENT AND PLANNING OF THE HEALTH SERVICE IN THE USSR/OASU "HEALTH"/

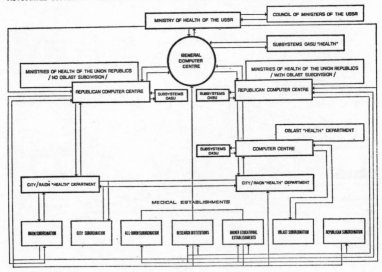

Fig. 8.

THREE ASPECTS OF IRREGULARITY IN BIOMEDICAL SCIENCE:

1. VARIATIONS IN NATURAL SCIENCES
2. VARIATIONS IN BIOMEDICAL RESEARCH FIELDS
3. VARIATIONS IN RESEARCH EFFORTS IN DIFFERENT COUNTRIES

THREE «BARRIERS» IN BIOMEDICAL RESEARCH:

1. INFORMATION BARRIER
2. METHODOLOGICAL BARRIER
3. SOCIAL & ETHICAL BARRIERS

Fig. 9a.

GRAPH OF THE OBJECTIVES OF OASU „HEALTH"

/ALL-UNION LEVEL/

FUNCTIONAL SUBSYSTEMS (1st order)

1. „CURE-PROPH"- MANAGEMENT OF THE CURATIVE AND PROPHYLACTIC SERVICE
2. „SANEPID"- MANAGEMENT OF THE SANITARY EPIDEMIOLOGICAL SERVICE
3. „PLANFIN"- MANAGEMENT OF THE PLANNING AND FINANCIAL ACTIVITIES
4. „PHARM"- PLANNING THE DRUG SUPPLY AND MANAGEMENT OF THE PHARMACY SERVICE
5. „MANPOWER"- PLANNING AND MANAGEMENT OF MANPOWER RESOURCES AND AN ACCOUNT OF SCIENTIFIC AND LEADING INSTITUTIONS
6. „MEDSTAT"- MEDICAL STATISTICS
7. „ASSMI"- A SYSTEM OF SCIENTIFIC MEDICAL AND MEDICO-TECHNOLOGICAL INFORMATION
8. „FNRI"- A FOND OF NORMATIVE REFERENCE INFORMATION

FUNCTIONAL SUBSYSTEMS (2nd order)

1. „CAPCONSTRUCT"- MANAGEMENT OF CAPITAL CONSTRUCTION
2. „MEDTECH"- MANAGEMENT OF INSTALLMENT SUPPLY AND MEDICAL TECHNICAL EQUIPMENT MAINTENANCE
3. „MATECHSUPPLY"- MANAGEMENT OF MATERIAL AND TECHNOLOGICAL SUPPLIES
4. „BOOK-ACCOUNTS"- SYSTEMS OF BOOK-ACCOUNTS AND CONTROL
5. „MEDSCIENCE"- MANAGEMENT AND COORDINATION OF SCIENTIFIC MEDICAL RESEARCH
6. OTHER SUBSYSTEMS

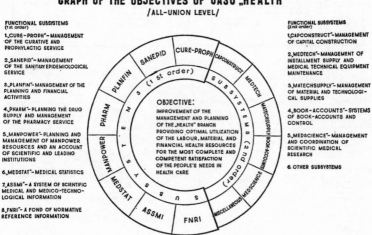

Fig. 9b.

PROJECTED DIRECTIONS AND PROBLEMS OF MEDICAL SCIENCE

LEVEL OF INVESTIGATION / PROBLEMS	CARDIO-VASCULAR DISEASE	CARCINOMA AND OTHER MALIGNANT NEOPLASMS	VIRAL INFECTIONS	BACTERIAL AND OTHER INFECTIONS	DISTURBANCES OF NUTRIT., METABOLISM, ENDOCRINE DISEASE	HEREDITARY AND CONGENITAL DISEASE	EFFECT OF DELETERIOUS ENVIRONMENTAL FACTORS
SOCIAL HYGIENE, PUBLIC HEALTH ORGANIZATION, SCIENCE MANAGEMENT	●	●	●	●	●	●	●
PSYCHOLOGY, BEHAVIORAL SCIENCES, PSYCHIATRY		●			●	●	●
INDIVIDUAL DEVELOPMENT OF THE ORGANISM AND AGE-RELATED PATHOLOGY	●	●			●	●	●
GENERAL AND SPECIAL IMMUNOLOGY		●	●	●	●	●	●
ORGANIZATION OF BIOLOGICAL SUSTEMS (INTEGRAL AND FUNCTIONAL)	●				●		●
MOLECULAR BIOLOGY, CELLULAR REPRODUCTION AND GENETICS		●	●	●	●	●	●

Fig. 10.

LONG-TERM PROGRAMME OF INTERNATIONAL COOPERATION IN CANCER RESEARCH

POSSIBILITY FACTORS:
RELATIVE PROGRAMME'S LIMITS
PRE-"BREAK-THROUGH" SITUATION IN CANCER RESEARCH AREAS
HISTORY OF CANCER RESEARCH COOPERATION
LARGE NATIONAL CANCER PROGRAMMES
BILATERAL & MULTILATERAL AGREEMENTS ON CANCER RESEARCH
GENERAL PUBLIC AND GOVERNMENTAL APPEAL & SUPPORT

POSSIBLE PROGRAMME'S BASIS:
UN RESOLUTION 1398 (XIY) ON INTERNAT. ENCOURAGEMENT OF SCIENT. RESEARCH IN CANCEROUS DISEASES (20.XI.59)
WHA. 26.61 (1973)
WHA. 27.63 (1974)
COOPERATIVE EFFORTS OF WHO (INCL. IACR), UCC AND NATIONAL INSTITUTIONS

INDISPENSABLE CONDITIONS FOR SUCCESS OF PROGRAMME:
1. FULL WILLINGNESS TO PARTICIPATE OF ALL COUNTRIES AND NATIONAL INSTITUTES. NO RESEARCH DICTATORSHIP.
2. CLEAR EVIDENCE OF ADVANTAGES OF PARTICIPATION IN PROGRAMME FOR NATIONAL INSTITUTES (ROUTINE REPORTING OF RESEARCH FINDINGS AND PRIORITIES, AND ACCESS OF PARTICIPANTS TO ALL RESULTS OF PROGRAMME.
3. SYSTEMATIC APPROACH TO CONSTRUCTION OF AN INFORMATION SYSTEM (FLEXIBLE USE OF COMPUTERS AND EFFECTIVE INTRODUCTION OF NEW DATA ON THE BASIS OF UNIFORM RECORDING OF RESEARCH SUBJECTS AND PLANS, THEIR METHODOLOGY AND RESULTS).

FACTORS FACILITATING NETWORK PLANNING AND IMPLEMENTATION OF PROGRAMME:
1. THE NETWORK DIAGRAM IS ESTABLISHED TENTATIVELY FOR 8-10 YEARS, AND NOT FOR DIRECTIVE PLANNING OF COMPONENTS OF PROGRAMME.
2. THE NETWORK DIAGRAM IS INTENDED NOT TO PREDICT FUTURE RESULTS, BUT TO REFLECT IN A ROUTINE WAY THE STATUS OF THE RESEARCH PROJECTS IN RELATION TO THE LONG-TERM GOALS.
3. THE NETWORK DIAGRAM IS INFORMATIONAL; IT DOES NOT CONSTITUTE THE BASIS FOR FINANCIAL, STAFFING OR OPERATIONAL DECISIONS (WHICH ARE THE PREROGATIVE OF THE NATIONAL INSTITUTIONS).

WHO 75045

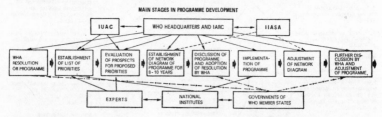

Fig. 11.

THE NATIONAL PATTERN OF HEALTH CARE AND
DELIVERY IN THE UNITED STATES AND ITS EFFECTS ON
THE EDUCATION, RECRUITMENT AND MIGRATION OF
PHYSICIANS

M. K. DuVAL
Arizona Medical Center, Tucson, Arizona, USA

ON JULY 4, 1776, the thirteen United Colonies representing Great
Britain in the western hemisphere declared their independence from
the rule of King George III and began operating as a Confederation
of states.

In the summer of 1787 representatives from twelve of these thirteen
states met in Philadelphia, in the state of Pennsylvania, to see if
they could further improve on the manner in which the new United
States of America were to be governed. Their deliberations culminated
in the production of a document which, over the next two years,
was ratified by the state Legislatures of nine of the states and thus
became the law of the land.

It is well to recognize that the Constitution that was adopted for
the United States speaks more to the form and structure of government rather than to a philosophy of government. Recognizing this,
the new Congress of the United States, as its first order of business,
urged the adoption of ten amendments to the Constitution. These
amendments were directed at the rights and privileges that the
people were to reserve unto themselves. Thus, the philosophy of
government in the United States, and the subsequent evolution of
the American people as a contemporary society, are perhaps more
accurately traceable to this 'Bill of Rights' rather than to the
Constitution itself.

If it is fair to ascribe the American way of life to its system of
recognizing the individual as supreme, then it is equally fair to
observe that among the principal weaknesses of this form of government is that it must expend a substantial portion of its energies in
the search for equity in reconciling opposing views. Thus, the
assignment of priorities, the allocation of the nation's resources,
and the development of centralized policies are inordinately difficult
exercises and lend credence to the view that the American society
is a laissez-faire enterprise that often seems deficient in having a
discrete purpose and an identifiable direction. It is within this
context that I have chosen to describe the national pattern of health

care and delivery in the United States and its effect on the education, recruitment and migration of physicians.

In most situations, prudence alone would deter me from oversimplifying my description of the American system for distributing medical services. However, because this audience is especially sophisticated, and the need for expediency in this short presentation is great, I will throw caution to the winds and describe American medicine as consisting of two principal components: a private sector that is self-determining and operates as a franchised monopoly; and a public sector whose primary mission is to meet those needs that either cannot or will not be met by the private sector. Let me start by describing the private sector.

As is true in most developing nations, the resevoir of professional knowledge with respect to the healing arts at the time of the birth of the United States was, for the most part, the exclusive property of those who practiced the healing arts. Medicine was not institutionalized in the United States at that time. Most medical knowledge was passed from one generation to the next by the direct instruction of one student by one physician; the circulation of medical knowledge through the printed and spoken word was greatly limited and institutions of higher education, with a few notable exceptions, did not constitute a part of the mainstream of medical knowledge. In 1847, individual practicing physicians joined together for the purpose of increasing their capacity to communicate with one another, advance medical knowledge, bring standards into the practice of medicine, and otherwise take such steps as were necessary to upgrade and strengthen their profession. Today, 127 years later, the American Medical Association still pursues those objectives and continues to serve as the most prominent voice representing the private sector of American medicine. Because of its relatively early arrival on the American scene, this association enjoyed the unique opportunity of fostering the further development of American medicine as an essentially private and self-determining profession essentially unchallenged in its supremacy in medical matters.

What do I mean by self-determining? In the United States, the medical profession is granted exclusive jurisdiction over the selection, examination and instruction of those who are to become physicians. It oversees the postgraduate training of those physicians who wish to become specialists. It certifies those who meet its standards and it has exclusive jurisdiction over medical licensure. Individual physicians are completely free to choose the town or city in which they will live and practice; they may select their own associates; affiliate with hospitals of their own choice; and otherwise participate in organizations that serve their own interests. Physicians serve as advisors to governmental agencies, dominate the field of health planning, and participate heavily in the decision-making ventures that culminate in the allocation of public resources in support of health efforts. Further, in the daily practice of medicine, physicians make all professional decisions, set their own fees, and organize the modalities by which health services are delivered; all of this without any external regulation.

Such freedom has, of course, permitted the development of a very strong profession. It has also made possible a great deal of experimentation and variety in the manner in which the private sector distributes health services. Physicians may work as individual solo practitioners or in small groups that take the form either of single discipline practices or multi-discipline group practices. Recently, some physicians have combined into larger organizations for the purpose of creating closed panels to render comprehensive services to large groups of citizens who choose to enroll as members. In many such instances the traditional fee for service mode of payment has been displaced by prepayment schemes.

As with the individual providers of medical care, institutional medicine in the United States is also strongly oriented to the private sector. Indeed, many of the individual institutions have so much capacity for self-determination that they, too, tend to operate independently of each other in such a way as to compete for the privilege of rendering services. The inevitable consequence of such an arrangement is to lead to an inordinate lack of co-ordination and an unnecessarily expensive duplication of facilities and physical resources such as nursing homes, community hospitals and specific treatment modalities such as radiation therapy and open heart surgery.

In summary then, American medicine is characterized by the high degree of freedom, autonomy and professional self-determination that are enjoyed by each of its practitioners and institutions, relatively free (at least until very recently) of external regulation and control.

Let me turn now to a brief description of the public sector of medicine in the United States. Briefly, there are three levels of governmental medicine, each of which tends to subserve a somewhat different function. At the most local level is the county, or in a few specific instances city, government. For the most part, local government assumes responsibility for providing both ambulatory and general medical and surgical hospital care for the poor, and it operates programs of preventive medicine and public health, including sanitation and environmental control.

The next level is state government. Until recently, when public financing of medical care began to assume increased prominence in the United States, the role of state government was primarily additive, or complementary, to the services provided by county government and found expression in the establishment of institutions and facilities for the care of individuals with chronic disabling diseases such as tuberculosis and mental illness. State governments participate in public health and preventive medicine programs. States also operate laboratories and are involved in sanitation and environmental control programs.

For approximately 150 years the Federal government has also been making a contribution to the American health industry but, until quite recently, its role was rather specific and directed at meeting the requirements of designated federal beneficiaries. In 1798, the Federal government created the United States Public Health Service and charged it with responsibility for providing medical services to sick and disabled seamen and protecting the nation's borders against the importation of diseases that were foreign to American soil. Over the succeeding years, the Federal government gradually undertook a somewhat broader public health responsibility by establishing closer relationships with state and local health departments for the purpose of controlling communicable diseases and improving sanitation. Next, it adopted programs to meet what it construed to be its obligations to provide medical services to specific beneficiaries such as the native-born American Indian, members of the armed forces and the veterans of America's wars. Programs for the care of these federal beneficiaries are still very prominent in Federal medicine today.

The establishment of the National Cancer Institute in 1937 opened a new era for the federal role in health because it offered direct federal support for biomedical research. This move culminated in the creation of the extramural programs of the National Institutes of Health, which programs supported research in the private sector. Almost simultaneously, the Federal government began moving more heavily into the field of regulation, food and drug inspections and control of the environment through programs designed to combat pollution of air and water. Even more recently, political and social pressures in the United States resulted in the development of federal programs designed to meet the health problems of particular population groups such as migrant farm workers, mothers and children among the poor, crippled children, those afflicted with alcoholism and drug abuse and the mentally ill.

Since the role of the U.S. government in health has become so complex in recent years, it might be helpful to clarify my description of this role by noting that the U.S. government now does five things. First, it has accepted an important responsibility for providing health services *directly* to certain specific beneficiaries. The government employs many thousands of physicians, dentists and other health personnel and operates hundreds of health care institutions for these purposes. The Department of Defense has a medical establishment that is now scattered throughout the world. The Veteran's Administration operates one of the world's largest closed-systems for the direct provision of health services to veterans. The U.S. Public Health Service dispenses care directly to merchant seamen, federal prisoners, members of the Coast Guard, and American Indians. Even at this time, the Public Health Service is experimenting with a National Health Service Corps which assigns physicians to render medical services to persons who live in geographically under-served areas.

Second, the Federal government provides health care *indirectly* through grants and contracts to private organizations and to state and local health departments. These units then provide health care to specific population groups such as migrant farm workers, the inner city poor, mothers and infants, crippled children, and others. Both the Veteran's Administration and the Department of Defense also have the capability for purchasing specific services from the local private sector so that they will not have to duplicate, un-necessarily, such services within their own systems.

Third, the Federal government has undertaken a major role in the development of health resources. The National Institutes of Health oversees the largest enterprise in the world in support of both basic and targeted biomedical research. The Health Resources Administration supports the production of traditional and new forms of health manpower and supports the construction of community hospitals through the federal Hill-Burton program.

Fourth, the Federal government has taken on a progressively increasing responsibility for quality control through the inspection and regulation of those instruments, devices and consumable supplies that constitute a part of the paraphernalia of the health industry and which are not otherwise controlled by the private sector. The Department of Agriculture now inspects and grades all meat and poultry products. The Food and Drug Administration reviews, inspects and regulates the flow of drugs; inspects the processing of foods and regulates the production of cosmetics. It also has responsibility for the regulation of hazardous substances and for radiological safety. The Federal government also monitors the purity of water and air.

Fifth, during the last two decades there has been a growing feeling in the United States that reasonable and convenient access to quality health services should be among the rights of the American people.

Public concern has now reached a point such that a national debate is underway as to how best to achieve such an objective as a matter of public policy. Because we have a medical profession that is intrinsically self-determining, and is thus in conflict with a public policy that would mandate coequal access to its services, the Federal government finds itself in the position of attempting to reconcile these competing objectives. Simply put, the government has two choices: using its extraordinary influence and resources to achieve reform of the traditional institutions for distributing health services, or else taking over control of the health industry. Perhaps because of our heritage, we have chosen, thus far, to pursue the first of these two alternate options. As a result, we have recently seen a plethora of new federal programs designed to encourage, indeed stimulate, modifications and reforms of the traditional American institutions as, for example, the Regional Medical Programs for cancer, heart, stroke and kidney disease; comprehensive health planning; experimental community health care delivery systems; emergency medical services programs; the development of health maintenance organizations; and the introduction of new methods for financing medical care, most notably the American Medicare and Medicaid systems.

Thus far, there has not been enough time to permit a proper evaluation of the impact such programs are having on the American health industry. The degree to which these programs are successful will, in all likelihood, determine whether the Federal government will adopt a national health insurance program or a National Health Service.

Let me now consider the effect that our national pattern of health care and delivery has on the education, recruitment and migration of physicians in the United States. As noted earlier, the reservoir of medical knowledge at the time of the birth of our nation was, for all practical purposes, limited to those persons who were actively engaged in the practice of the healing arts since there were almost no institutions offering formal programs in medical education in the United States at that time. Medical practitioners of that era drew their knowledge from three principal sources: that which was already being practiced by native Americans; that which came primarily from Spain and accompanied the migration into the United States through Mexico; and the northern European medicine that arrived on American shores through immigration. This medical knowledge was forwarded into each succeeding generation either from father to son or, in some instances, by a preceptorship system in which a young and interested student apprenticed himself to a practicing physician.

Beginning in the eighteenth and nineteenth centuries, physicians who were interested in medical education formed partnerships and developed proprietary schools of medicine that featured lectures and demonstrations with a minimum of either basic science teaching or opportunity for clinical experience. Simultaneously, a few universities like Johns-Hopkins (which had been consciously modeled after the scientific, sophisticated German universities), began to offer medical education of a much higher quality such that the contrasts and variabilities in medical education were very great; so great, in fact, that the Carnegie Foundation for the Advancement of Teaching sponsored a country-wide survey of medical education in 1908, culminating in the publication of the 'Flexner Report' in 1910. The effect of this report was to close most of the proprietary schools of medicine and restore jurisdiction for medical education to the universities. It had the further effect of introducing educational standards for medical schools, reemphasizing the scientific base of medical education and creating the full-time system of salaried medical faculty capable of undertaking clinical teaching in the environment of a teaching hospital.

It has taken all of the ensuing sixty years for us to measure the full impact of the Flexner Report on medicine in the United States. Certainly a substantial portion of the extraordinary advances that American medicine has made can be attributed to the changes that followed the Flexner Report. At the same time, many of America's most serious problems in medicine are also traceable to the impact of the Report.

Consider, for example, that after medical education was restored to the university campus there followed a marked increase in the number of persons who devoted their professional career to medical education. Because these teaching physicians were not primarily engaged in traditional medical practice, the base for their clinical instruction of medical students became the hospitalized patient. Further, as their individual expertise increased these teachers were increasingly called upon by practitioners in the field for assistance in the management of difficult and complex medical cases. The increasing concentration of complicated medical problems in the teaching setting stimulated medical faculty members to devote a substantial part of their time to medical research. The beneficial impact on society of competent medical research, and the progressive elimination of certain medical problems traceable to medical advances, were promptly recognized by governmental representatives and a massive investment of federal funds was undertaken in the further support of medical research. This large investment, mostly absorbed by American medical faculties, generated such an explosion of medical knowledge that individual members of medical faculties could no

longer encompass but a small part of the newly expanding knowledge. These faculty members thus began to compartmentalize
themselves and their knowledge in specialty disciplines and
organizations. As each faculty member narrowed the scope of his
particular expertise and interests, and since medical schools were still
awarding a universal doctor of medicine degree, the size of medical
faculties had to be increased and medical schools had to seek more
resources to support their enterprises.

Unfortunately, this mode of operation did not permit a parallel
increase in undergraduate medical student enrollments. This situation
was aggravated by the heightening of public expectations that had
derived from the new advances in medicine such that student
demand for the study of medicine increased out of proportion to the
capacity of our medical schools to admit them. This caused a type of
competition for admission to medical school that we had not previously seen and created a new set of problems for which we have
not yet found an answer. Many of our students migrated to other
countries for this education. Meanwhile, medical schools found it
necessary to create committees whose sole function was to screen
and select, from among hundreds of applicants, those who were to
be admitted. Objective criteria that depended upon scholastic records
and a proven aptitude for taking tests were developed to such a
high order that the students who were ultimately selected for the
study of medicine tended to become scientific counterparts and
replications of the medical school faculties themselves. Such students,
upon entering the environment of the contemporary American
medical school, reinforced the movement toward sub-specialism in
American medicine and, being trained in the research-oriented and
highly specialized environment that characterized the American
medical school, resulted in the production of physicians who bore
little resemblance to their medical ancestors.

On leaving the medical school environment, such students either
entered high level medical administration, medical research or
graduate medical education so that they could practice their specialty
after the model of their instructors. This produced a marked fall
in the production of primary care physicians and an offsetting
increase in the production of highly specialized physicians. On
entering the world of medical practice, it was perhaps inevitable that
such physicians would seek to establish their practices in settings that
bore some resemblance to the setting in which they had been trained;
in other words, in urban and metropolitan areas where good hospital
facilities were available and where associations with similarly
trained physicians were possible. As older physicians, many of whom
were serving in rural and other geographically underserved areas,

retired from practice or died they were not replaced, and the increasing concentration of highly specialized physicians in urban-metropolitan areas of the United States created an imbalance which is now so serious as to constitute a topic of national concern.

Two elements have further exacerbated this situation. First, as already noted, the continuing rise of the American population without a concomitant increase in the production of physicians has made us deeply conscious of the possibility that we now have a true shortage of physicians in the United States. To some extent, this discrepancy has been offset both by the marked increase in productivity of each physician and, more recently, by the increased productivity that has been possible through the use of physician assistants and other physician extenders. Unfortunately, even this gain in individual productivity is more apparent than real because of the growth in the number of physicians who have narrowed the scope of their practices such that they may concentrate their efforts solely on those areas of medicine that are based on technological advance and, as a consequence, are of service to a smaller portion of the population.

Second, because of the relative shrinkage in numbers of physicians, and because of the introduction of new federal and state instruments for financing medical care, physicians have tended to migrate toward practice settings that are economically rewarding and that assure them appropriate compensation for their services. Thus, while it has been the intense increase in specialization that has mitigated against the migration of physicians into geographically underserved and rural areas, it has been the new methods of finance and the appeal of adequate compensation that have discouraged the migration of physicians into those high density urban settings where so many of America's poorer citizens must necessarily reside.

The contemporary American dilemma can thus be summarized as follows. American medicine is credited with having made an extraordinary contribution to the expansion of the scientific and technological basis of medical practice. These advances have had the paradoxical effect of whetting the American appetite for universal access to everything that medicine can make available at precisely the time that the dynamics of American medical education and practice appear to be moving in the opposite direction. One might say, then, that the stage is currently set for a major contest in the United States; a contest between the traditional right of the American medical profession to be free and self-determining and the countervailing right of the American people to have equitable access to the services of that profession. How this contest will be resolved remains uncertain.

Chapter 14

THE PROVISION OF MEDICAL CARE IN HOSPITALS AND ITS EFFECT ON EDUCATION

R. H. EBERT and T. COLTON
Harvard Medical School, Boston, USA

UNITED STATES medicine has had some remarkable successes, many of them associated with American medical schools and teaching hospitals. But there have been failures and there is a rising tide of public criticism which will almost certainly alter our medical care system as well as our approach to medical education. Two failures which relate both directly and indirectly to our educational system are : (1) the maldistribution of physicians among the medical specialists, and (2) the geographic maldistribution of physicians in the United States. It might be argued that medical education has little or no responsibility for the geographic location of physicians in practice but it is possible to show that the way in which physicians are trained does influence their choice of where to practice. And I hasten to add that I am including graduate physicians' education as an integral part of our medical educational system.

Too little attention has been paid to the key role of house staff—namely, interns, residents and clinical fellows—in our teaching hospitals. Their involvement in both teaching and patient care is central to our understanding of our system of medical education. Indeed, our reliance on the services of house staff for the care of the hospitalized patient is important in understanding the reason why large community hospitals have recruited substantial numbers of foreign medical graduates.

The Evolution of the Teaching Hospital

The report of the Carnegie Foundation for the Advancement of Teaching authored by Abraham Flexner (1910)[3] had many effects but only one is germane to this discussion, namely, its impact on the teaching hospital. The report urged that teaching hospitals become integral parts of universities, that full-time clinical faculties should be developed, and that clinical faculty members should devote their efforts to research and teaching rather than to their lucrative private practices. What evolved was not precisely what Flexner had in mind, but profound changes did occur, and for over half a century the Flexnerian philosophy has been the dominant influence in medical education.

No single prototype of the 'teaching hospital' developed since a number of quite different kinds of hospitals were inaugurated into the educational system. But all developed full-time faculties, to a greater or lesser degree, all emphasized research and teaching and, as we shall see, all became deeply involved in the postgraduate training of physicians. What kinds of hospitals are we talking about? The list includes voluntary hospitals, city or county hospitals, university hospitals, some private and some state owned, Veterans Administration hospitals, and more recently, some so-called community hospitals.

For the purpose of this discussion, it is convenient to group large voluntary hospitals with city and county hospitals because both were originally created to care for the sick-poor and both had a profound influence on the postgraduate education of physicians. The Massachusetts General Hospital, for example, founded in 1811, was a voluntary hospital originally conceived of as a place where the poor of Boston could be cared for when they were ill, it being accepted that the more affluent citizens of the city could receive better care at home. The founders also expressed the view that the hospital should be used for teaching, since care was provided without charge and therefore patients could hardly object to being used for the instruction of physicians in training. The Boston City Hospital was founded in 1864 with similar purposes in mind, and both became distinguished teaching hospitals. They diverged, of course, when in 1919 the Massachusetts General Hospital built its first private pavillion for the care of paying patients, but for many years they retained certain important similarities. In both hospitals the teaching of medical students was conducted entirely on the charity wards and both developed programs for the postgraduate training of physicians which delegated substantial—indeed, often complete— responsibility for the care of patients to the house staff, namely, interns and residents. These hospitals were not unique, and had their counterpart in other major cities in the United States.

The 'university hospital,' and here reference is made to the hospital owned or operated by the university, evolved in a rather different manner, or to be more accurate, in different manners since two distinct types developed. One was the state-owned hospital operated by the state medical school, and the other was the private university hospital owned and operated by the university. State university hospitals were built specifically as teaching institutions and since they were publicly funded, it was usually stated that they were not to compete with private practitioners but were to serve as a source of referral on a state-wide basis for physicians in practice. Of course, it did not work out that way. Some became heavily engaged in the private practice of medicine, some were used as a resource for the medically indigent in the state, and some became the equivalent of the 'city hospital' for the local community. Usually there was no sharp separation between 'private' and 'public' patients and the full time faculty usually assumed primary responsibility for the care of patients. In other words, the house staff was more closely supervised as a rule than in the city hospital or the charity wards of the voluntary hospital.

The privately owned 'university hospital' evolved in a somewhat similar manner, although here the hypothetical constraint on competition with the private practitioner was absent. Some developed with entirely full time staffs, some with a mix of full and part time, but all became heavily engaged in the cure of the paying patient. Often no distinction was made between the charity and the paying patient, and as in the state university hospital the house officer was given less direct responsibility than in the first two types of hospitals. These hospitals became very much specialty orientated and often the services were divided by subspecialties rather than as the more general medical and surgical ward of the voluntary hospital or the city hospital.

Until the end of World War II, Veterans Administration hospitals were little more than domiciliary facilities, and were not used for teaching by American medical schools. Beginning in 1946, however, there was a massive reform of these hospitals and an important part of the strategy of reform was to develop a close working relationship with medical schools. This helped in the recruitment of staff since many able physicians were attracted by the opportunity to have full-time faculty appointments in affiliated medical schools, and it also enabled V.A. hospitals to recruit house staff. The *quid pro quo* for the medical school was a teaching hospital paid for by the federal government (oftimes new and built adjacent to the medical school), a teaching facility for medical students taught by faculty selected by the medical school, but on the federal payroll, and another resource for house staff. As a matter of policy, admission to a Veterans Administration hospital for a non-service connected illness required evidence of medical indigency, and while this policy was never strictly followed it did permit the use of all patients for teaching and also allowed a substantial delegation of responsibility for patient care to house staff. Since Veterans Administration hospitals served a predominantly male population, they were not suitable as a total teaching environment for interns and residents with the result that most university affiliated Veterans Administration hospitals became integral parts of house staff programs that used at least one other teaching hospital.

In recent years some large community hospitals have been used for teaching without becoming fully integrated into the medical school teaching complex. The attraction to the hospital is the opportunity to recruit house staff. These hospitals, however, do not represent an important part of the teaching environment.

Specialty Training

In the early part of this century the majority of medical graduates went immediately into practice after medical school or took only one year of internship. It gradually became customary for all graduates wishing to practice to take a year of internship and in the 1920's and 1930's, specialty training became more popular. Such training, however, tended to be concentrated in major medical centers and it was not uncommon for physicians to specialize only after some years in general practice.

Following World War II the pattern changed rapidly and specialization immediately after graduation became the rule rather than the exception. The recruitment of house staff became a major preoccupation for herds of university clinical departments and it was during this period that specialty training programs came to be such an important part of the teaching environment.

Even before World War II, subspecialization in fields such as cardiology, gastroenterology and endocrinology had become an important part of the academic scene, but usually subspecialization grew out of the research interests of the academic physician rather than a desire to practice a subspecialty. The development of training programs in the various specialties by the National Institutes of Health during the 1950's and 1960's accelerated a trend already present in teaching hospitals and the broad fields of internal medicine and surgery became increasingly subdivided. Obviously, the purpose of such programs was the training of clinical investigators, but many trainees became practitioners rather than investigators and the subspecialist became an accepted model for the practice of medicine.

Prior to World War II many medical school graduates sought internship in community hospitals and it was customary to choose a hospital in a community where the graduate wished to practice, since internship was the first step in acquiring staff privileges in the hospital. Immediately following World War II, many community hospitals expanded their programs to include residency training and the influx of physicians who were veterans seeking specialty training plus medical school graduates enabled community hospitals to recruit the graduates of American medical schools.

Beginning in the early 1950's community hospitals found it more and more difficult to recruit the graduates of American schools into residency programs and at the same time residency programs in university teaching hospitals became increasingly popular. There were a number of reasons for this trend which continues to the present day. First of all, medical school graduates became more mobile and no longer looked for opportunities for training either near their homes or even where they wished to practice. They realized that excellent training could be just as important in acquiring staff privileges at a community hospital as was being a graduate of the community hospital's own training program. Indeed, it might be more important to come from elsewhere if one brought a needed subspecialty skill to the community hospital. Another important reason was the degree of responsibility given the intern and resident. Since almost all patients in community hospitals were private, far less direct responsibility was given the intern and resident as compared with the teaching hospital with its charity ward tradition. Most medical school graduates sought training programs which provided the maximum responsibility to the house officer. The strength of the teaching hospital in the various subspecialties as compared with the community hospital provided an additional incentive. Even the resident who did not wish to become a subspecialist felt that he could learn more from the expert than the generalist, and the environment of the teaching hospital was such that the resident felt that he was in the vanguard of modern medicine —as indeed he was. In the 1950's and early 1960's, the community hospital could not at times attract interns and residents by paying more than the teaching hospitals, but this pay differential ceased to exist after the mid-1960's when all house officers began to receive something approaching a living wage.

Community hospitals were interested in the recruitment of interns and residents not because of any social sense of responsibility, but for very practical reasons. House officers provided relatively cheap labor and were important not only in providing care for hospitalized patients, but also in manning emergency rooms and hospital Out-Patient Departments. As it became more difficult to recruit graduates of American schools, efforts were made to recruit graduates of foreign medical schools, often from Asia. It is important to note, however, that teaching hospitals as well came to rely heavily on foreign medical graduates in those specialties such as pathology and anesthesiology, which were less popular with American graduates. Again, the motivation was patient care and not teaching. *Table 1*

(p. 154) illustrates this point. In 1960, among a total of 20,609 house officers in teaching hospitals, 3,402 or 16.5% were foreign medical graduates. In 1970, the number of foreign medical graduates in teaching hospitals had increased to 11,587 and constituted 26.9% of all such house officers. In nonteaching hospitals in 1960, foreign medical graduates numbered 6,055 or 38.3% of all house staff. In 1970, although the number of foreign medical graduates in non-teaching hospitals decreased in absolute number to 4,695, they represented proportionately a larger share of all such house officers, namely 60.8%. Note that between 1960 and 1970 total house staff in teaching hospitals more than doubled; in contrast, total house staff in nonteaching hospitals decreased by more than half.

Reliance of Teaching Hospital on House Staff

This increase in the number of house officers in teaching hospitals represents both an expansion in the number of teaching hospitals and the number of house officers in each hospital. There is little doubt that the teaching hospital has become heavily dependent on house staff for the provision of care to both hospitalized and ambulatory patients. In large part, this is due to the increasingly complex technology of medicine and the extension of what it is possible to do for the sick patient. The advent of open heart surgery, for example, required in addition to the surgical team, a very considerable expansion of the duties of cardiologists and radiologists and the resulting demand for additional manpower expanded the number of trainees in these fields. Similarly, the feasibility of renal transplantation led to the development of a new field of medical subspecialization, namely, renal dialysis. So much of what happens in medicine is palliative rather than curative that advances in technology usually mean an increase in manpower requirements rather than a decrease, and this is reflected in the demand for house officers. It is not generally realized that interns, residents and fellows represent fifteen percent of the total pool of practicing physicians in the United States and in some fields such as internal medicine and surgery they represent one quarter of all the physicians in the specialties (Figure 1, p. 155).

The Teaching Environment

For the past two decades, curriculum change has provided a major diversion for American medical faculties. There has been endless discussion of the best way to teach the basic sciences, the pros and cons of integrated teaching, the virtue of elective time, and the importance of early clinical experience. Curiously, there has been almost no general discussion of how clinical teaching is done and yet it is the keystone of medical education in the United States. It is also heavily dependent on interns, residents and fellows.

If one were to try to characterize the nature of clinical teaching in the simplest terms, one would say that the medical student learns by becoming a member of the 'ward team'. There are many variants of the ward team, but in essence the members are the 'visit'—a faculty member who for a month or two is the senior member of the team— a junior resident (sometimes accompanied by a senior resident), two interns, and two or more medical students. The medical students and interns 'work up' all of the patients and provide the day to day care under the supervision of the residents and all are ultimately accountable to the visit who conducts the formal teaching rounds and quizzes both medical student and house staff on what they have done and why. Obviously, there are many variations of the ward team depending on the particular specialty and the character of the teaching hospital, but by and large, the medical student learns by direct involvement in the care of the patient rather than by demonstration and much of what he learns is taught by the house staff. If the house staff is of poor quality and disinterested the teaching will be poor, whereas the student will learn rapidly if the house staff is responsible and concerned both for the care of the patient and the quality of the teaching environment.

Recently, the Harvard Medical School completed a rather elaborate study of how both faculty and house staff spend their time and the results are revealing. The study was headed by Dr. Ivan J. Fahs, a medical sociologist. Very briefly, the methodology consisted of data collection by a self-reporting questionnaire format. A whole day— midnight to midnight—was defined as the reporting unit. The entire full-time faculty was asked to respond on three separate randomly selected days, whereas fifty percent samples of part-time faculty and those in training status were taken and asked to report only one randomly selected day. Further details on the methodology may be obtained elsewhere (Colton, Fahs and Feldman 1974)[1].

Table 2 (p. 154) gives the number of faculty in each category together with the number in training status. The faculty of Harvard Medical School includes two full-time categories—academic full time and clinical full time. Clinical full-time faculty spends a larger proportion of time with patient care and less time in research activities than the academic full-time faculty. Both are expected to teach. Training status includes interns, residents and postdoctoral fellows. The table shows the number of questionnaires distributed, the number and percent returned, and in the last column, the mean

hours of professional activity per week in each category based on a
52-week year.

Figure 2 (p. 155) gives the percent of time in teaching and all
activities related to teaching by status in the clinical faculty and
those in training status at the Harvard Medical School. This percent
of activity includes time spent in the preparation of lectures,
laboratories and demonstrations, as well as actual contact with
students.

For all categories of faculty except part-time, a considerable portion
of total professional time was spent in teaching activities, roughly
about thirty percent.

In Figure 3 (p. 156), superimposed on total teaching of any kind
are the following subclassifications of teaching: (a) teaching with
students present, (b) teaching with Harvard medical or dental students
present, and finally, (c) teaching with Harvard medical or dental
students only present. It may be seen that for each category of
faculty the large majority of total teaching time was spent in the
presence of some type of students. In turn, when students were
present during teaching, a good portion of such time—at least more
than half—involved the presence of Harvard medical or dental
students. Those in training status spent the largest portion of their
time in teaching activities with Harvard medical or dental students
present—nearly one-fifth of their total professional activity. Academic
full-time and clinical full-time faculty spent somewhat less time
in teaching with Harvard medical or dental students present,
namely, about one-tenth of their total professional time; for part-
time faculty this teaching category accounted for six percent of
their total time.

The last teaching subclassification in Figure 3 indicates that in
each category of faculty little time was spent—roughly two percent of total professional activity—in teaching with only Harvard
medical or dental students present to the exclusion of other types
of students. Thus, when a faculty member was involved in teaching
with Harvard medical and/or dental students present, usually other
students were present as well. This indicates that with the clinical
teaching activities that were directed towards Harvard's medical
and dental students, other students—mostly house staff—profited
as well by being present during such activity.

Figure 4 (p. 157) indicates by faculty category the percentage of
total professional time that respondents classified as involving patient
care. Part-time faculty spent the largest portion of their time,
seventy percent, in patient care while training status faculty spent
nearly three-fifths of their time in such activity. The clinical full-
time faculty expended more than half their total professional effort

in patient care while academic full-time faculty spent considerably less time, only about thirty percent in patient care. The latter two figures provide empirical justification for the administrative designation of the two distinct faculty categories of academic full-time and clinical full-time.

Figure 5 (p. 158) superimposes on patient care the proportion of time spent in teaching. One important facet of the study methodology was that respondents could characterize their activities with overlapping classifications. Thus, they were able to designate that a particular activity involved *both* teaching and patient care. It may be seen in Figure 5 that the joint category of teaching and patient care accounted for a considerable portion of total professional activity—about one-fifth for clinical full-time and training status faculty and roughly one-eighth for academic full-time and part-time faculty. It is also evident in Figure 5 that, except for academic full-time faculty, more time was spent in teaching associated with patient care than in teaching not associated with patient care. Even with academic full-time faculty, teaching in combination with patient care accounted for almost half of all teaching activity.

In summary, the results of this study reveal that for Harvard's clinical faculty:

1. A substantial proportion of time is spent in teaching and activities related to teaching.
2. When students are present during teaching activities, most of the time Harvard medical or dental students number among those present.
3. Generally, other students profit from teaching aimed at Harvard medical and dental students. When teaching occurs with Harvard medical or dental students present, almost always there are other students present as well.
4. A substantial portion of teaching activity occurs in conjunction with other activities; in particular, the majority of teaching time is spent in teaching combined with patient care.

Social Forces Which May Change the System

The teaching hospital provides the single most important part of the teaching environment for medical students and it is evident that the program for interns, residents and fellows are an integral part of the environment. What has evolved has been a remarkably successful educational experience. Students learn by active participation in patient care, but are under the constant critical scrutiny of both house staff and faculty. Students have the opportunity to learn about 'their patients' from an impressive array of consultants and again, the consulting team includes faculty and house staff. One can only conclude that any sudden change in the pattern of house staff training would profoundly affect the education of medical students.

All medical education in the United States is heavily dependent on public funds and therefore is vulnerable to changing government policy, particularly at the federal level. But the most vulnerable part of the system is the teaching hospital for it is subject to influences on both the education and patient care systems. A brief review of the social forces which can influence teaching hospitals will demonstrate this point.

1. *Payment mechanisms.* Most people agree that some kind of national insurance will be legislated in the United States in the near future. This will extend further the insurance coverage of United States citizens and will probably eliminate the so-called medically indigent patient. By itself, this change will not materially alter the teaching environment. Most teaching services have successfully adapted to a system which more and more requires the identification of a 'private physician' for the insured patient, without substantial change in the responsibility delegated to house staff. The impact would be profound, however, if there were a change in the reimbursement formula to teaching hospitals and inadequate funds were available for the support of house staff. For example, if the decision were made to allocate the cost of the time house staff spends teaching medical students to medical education rather than patient care, it could alter the system.

2. *Federal funding* of biomedical research, research training and medical education has influenced the way in which the clinical teaching environment has evolved. Recent changes in federal policy directed toward the funding of training programs in clinical departments has already modified the environment and the potential impact is even greater.

3. It was noted earlier that the American public is increasingly critical of both medical education and medical practice. The public is not so much concerned with the cost of medical care or the pros and cons of national health insurance as it is with the availability of physician services. One major concern is the great difficulty experienced by the ordinary citizen in finding a family physician and another is the almost total lack of medical services in some communities, particularly those that are rural. The Congress is well aware of these criticisms and Senator Kennedy's staff has been rewriting the health manpower legislation to do something about the maldistribution of physicians among the specialties as well as the

geographic maldistribution of physicians. The Senator's staff is well aware of the medical school-teaching hospital's involvement in this problem. They know that the present orientation of the teaching hospital is toward the specialties of medicine and that there are few opportunities for the student to participate in family practice or primary care. They are also aware that physicians trained in large urban hospitals oriented toward the specialties are unlikely to seek practice opportunities in small towns or rural communities.

It is quite possible that there will be regulation of the number of physicians allowed to enter the various medical specialties and that there will be the usual 'carrot-stick' approach to the training of more family physicians or primary care physicians. How this is done could profoundly affect the teaching hospital. There is no reason why the best of what has been created for the clinical teaching of students cannot be adapted to the training of more primary care physicians. But if the change is too abrupt and done without regard to the very real contributions of the 'ward team approach' to the teaching of clinical medicine, much of what has been accomplished by United States teaching hospitals over several decades could be dissipated.

4. Teaching hospitals have come to be viewed as a resource for the local community and are under increasing pressure to provide a total range of medical care for the local citizens.

5. The studies of Funkenstein (1974)[4] have revealed how little the medical school influences students in their attitudes toward medicine and their choice of careers. An increasing number of students are interested in careers in primary care and family medicine, but feel frustrated because of the lack of opportunity for training in the major teaching hospitals.

Conclusion

The interlocking of medical education with patient care at the clinical level is very close. Anything which alters the way in which care is provided in our teaching hospitals and specifically the future role of house staff in patient care will profoundly influence the education of the medical student. There is evidence to suggest that some substantial changes in the role of teaching hospitals may occur and this in turn will change the educational environment for medical students.

Bibliography

1. Colton, T., Fahs, I. J. and Feldman, C. S. (1974) *Unpublished manuscript.*
2. Ebert, R. H. (1973) *Sci. Amer.* 229, 139-148.
3. Flexner, A. (1910) *Medical Education in the United States and Canada: A Report to the Carnegie Foundation for the Advancement of Teaching.* New York, Bulletin No. 4.
4. Funkenstein, D. H., *An Overview of Seventeen Years of Research on Medical Students and Their Career Choices 1958-1974.* Proceedings of the Conference on Career Development of Physicians, Association of American Medical Colleges, June 17-19, 1974, Washington, D.C. (in press), 1974.
5. *Medical Education in the United States* (1973) J.A.M.A. 26, 935.

TABLE I

Number and percent of foreign medical graduates among house officers in hospitals affiliated with medical schools and in nonteaching hospitals, United States, 1960 and 1970 (from Ebert, 1974).

	Year	Total House Officers	Foreign Medical Graduates No.	%
Hospitals affiliated with medical schools:	1960	20,609	3,402	16.5
	1970	43,043	11,587	26.9
Nonteaching hospitals:	1960	15,829	6,055	38.3
	1970	7,724	4,695	60.8

TABLE II

Number of faculty, number of study questionnaires distributed and returned, and mean hours of professional activity per week by status, clinical faculty*, Havard Medical School, 1971-72.

Status	Number of Faculty	Study Questionnaires Distributed	Returned %	Mean Hours of Professional Activity Per week
Academic full time (AFT)	428	1,075	992 (92.2)	53.5
Clinical full time (CFT)	501	1,316	1,222 (92.9)	50.0
Part time (PT)	1,396	685	593 (86.6)	45.8
Training (TS)	1,050	504	403 (80.0)	49.3
Total clinical faculty	3,377	3,580	3,210 (89.7)	

* Includes all appointees of clinical departments.

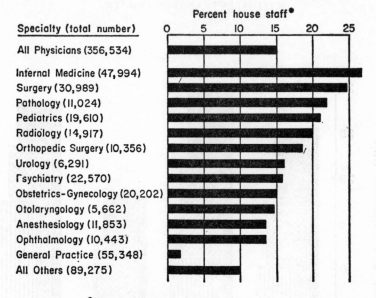

Figure 1. Percent physicians who are house staff by specialty, United States, 1972.

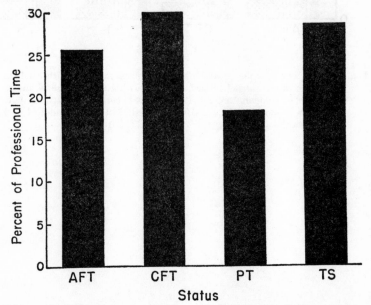

Figure 2. Percent of time in teaching and all activities related to teaching by status, clinical faculty, Harvard Medical School, 1971–72. (abbreviations as in Table 2, p. 154)

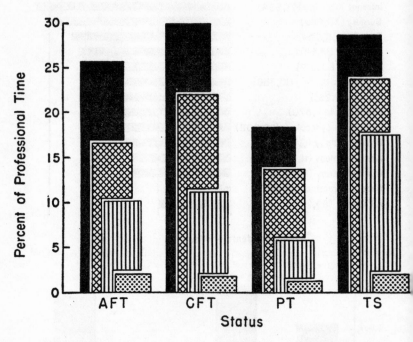

Figure 3. Percent of time in teaching (solid bar), teaching with students present (cross-hatched bar), teaching with Harvard medical and/or dental students present (vertical-lined bar) and teaching with *only* Harvard medical and/or dental students present (dotted bar), clinical faculty, Harvard Medical School, 1971–72.

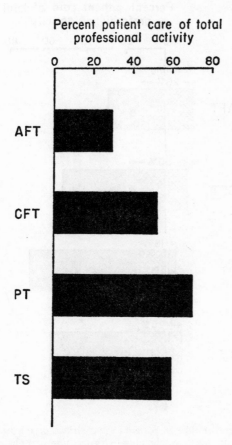

Figure 4. Percent of time in patient care, clinical faculty, Harvard Medical School, 1971–72.

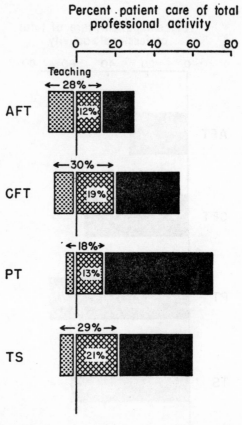

Figure 5. Percent of time in patient care exclusive of teaching (solid bar), patient care in combination with teaching (cross-hatched bar) and teaching exclusive of patient care (dotted bar), clinical faculty, Harvard Medical School, 1971–72.

Chapter 15

THE CHANGING ORGANIZATION OF HEALTH CARE IN THE UNITED STATES

E. W. SAWARD
School of Medicine and Dentistry, University of Rochester, N.Y., USA

MANY NATIONS appear to have a consistent policy in regard to health services for their citizens and have maintained such policies for significant periods of time. In general these policies are recent developments of this century and for many countries, of the last decades. However, fundamental roots of such policies may be perceived much further into the past. While there is usually no homogeneous cultural attitude about any policy, the consensus derives from advocacy of different opinions and the consistency of some expressions as central values.

The United States has undergone significant changes in the financing and structure of its health services in the past decade. There is every evidence that further major changes are now occurring and within a few years some form of National Health Insurance will become a reality. It is then quite likely that still further changes will come ever more rapidly. One would assume that from the present degree of change and the expectation of imminent further change that there might be an overall policy formulated to lead this evolution; or, if not a single policy, one might expect that the two opposing political parties might each have a single but differing policy. Further, that if neither the administration leadership had a policy, nor the opposing political parties, perhaps the entrenched bureaucracy through high-level civil servants would have a consistent policy for which they would try to gain acceptance. It is apparent that none of these suppositions is true. Dr. Charles Edwards, America's highest health official, recently stated—'There has never been a real federal health strategy with meaningful priorities.' (American Medical News, 1974)

There are, of course, various fragments and pieces of policy that have various advocates. But if one looks at the last decade or even the last three or four years, one cannot discern very much consistency even in regard to the pieces. There are almost no long-tenured, high-level civil servants in the field. The bureaucracy has been reorganized seven times in the last decade in an attempt to cope with the vast growth of health funding, and the turnover has been extreme and persons at high level have seldom been in their positions for more than a very few years. There appears to be no institutional memory in the bureaucracy and, whatever had been decided in the past as a rational approach, seems to have been forgotten, and policy determination appears to restart from a clean slate.

A health crisis was proclaimed by President Nixon five years ago with the statement that 'chaos would ensue if medical care was not reorganized'. It has not been reorganized and it is very difficult to discern any significant differences from the prevailing situation of five years ago. It is even difficult to discern whether there is as much disaffection today as he perceived then. Attention has been diverted to other areas of political concern, but with continued reaffirmation for desired reform in health affairs. There is, thus, no such thing as a unified federally sponsored national health policy and in fact there never has been. Of course, this is not intent to prejudge that there never will be. It is true that some consider this situation deplorable but on reflection it is in many ways charateristically American.

The attitudes and institutions concerned with medical care in the early history of the United States reflect its origin as a British colony. The 'sick poor' were a county public responsibility, hence, the county hospital. Merchant seamen, armed forces, and veterans were cared for by national government in categorical institutions reminiscent of Chelsea. But for the great majority of citizens health services were in the private domain, paid on a fee basis. The hospitals were private, independent philanthropies. Much of this heritage remains today and remains a factor shaping present policy.

America has moved but recently from the 'frontier ethic' where each person was largely responsible for his own enterprise and welfare. Many now see the central government becoming the instrument for such welfare, but the central government's official position appears to be that while it is responsible for much in the way of general policy and standards, it is the responsibility of local government to implement action for the welfare of the citizens. This concept is inherent in the current concept of 'general and special revenue sharing', whereby federal tax funds are redistributed to state and local government for decision as to use. Superficially this interplay might be seen as being far removed from health and relating only to political science. However, there is no question that health services, health financing, and health policy have been politicized, and these general concepts of our society affect health as but one of a spectrum of special concerns shaping policy.

Before we describe where we may possibly be going as a nation in this search of health policy, it seems well to review very briefly how we got where we are. The first deliberate event in the evolution of a national health policy in America is the Flexner Report of 1910. This was a study conducted under the sponsorship of a private foundation and its impact on the medical profession was perfectly timed to be a leading position that could be widely agreed upon. The Flexner Report clearly saw that medicine was changing from a profession whose abilities largely were those of caring for illness to one whose potential was for curing illness. In other words, 1910 in America was very good timing to forecast the rapid development of science and technology in medicine, and to appropriately change the nature of the institutions that educated physicians.

This belief in science and technology became ever more widespread with the passage of time. In America the belief in science and technology, reemphasized by governmental programs to create nuclear energy and to place man on the moon, has become a dominant cultural attribute, perhaps as widespread as any particular religion. The medical profession may overstate its technical power but the public believes it has the ability to perform even its overstated objectives. Miracles have been represented from the profession through the press to the public so frequently that the public expects miracles; and as the Congress reflects public sentiment, it sometimes believes that it is possible to legislate them. This cultural ambiance in regard to science and technology in medicine is one of the principal factors now shaping health policy.

As the result of a study conducted by another private philanthropy in the period 1927–1932, a report from the 'Committee on the Costs of Medical Care' produced a health policy of a scope and rationality that remains as relevant today as it was 40 years ago. This called for universal entitlement to health care in the United States through prepayment mechanisms, and the deliberate organization of health services in an integrated fashion through group practices and other means so that all would have access to health services without barrier and in a rational way. Unfortunately, this brilliant report had little effect on the American public and was vigorously opposed by the organized American medical profession, so that while it remains a milestone in policy formulation, its influence was only a shadow of what it should have been. There was an abortive attempt to partially implement it in the original Social Security Law of 1935. A section was written to provide such eligibility for health services of all the working population. However, in the enactment of the law, the section was dropped under the influence of special interest groups, including the organized medical profession, who felt such provision would be adverse to their interests.

Another attempt at National Health Insurance was made in that

rather unique period of reform that immediately followed World
War II when the spirit of equality and fraternity seemed to possess
many nations, however briefly. President Truman strongly advocated
such a program but, after several years, it was defeated largely due
to the efforts of the organized medical profession and the private
insurance industry. Organized labor had strongly backed this
approach but, upon its defeat and the ruling of the Supreme Court
that health benefits were a legitimate item of collective negotiation
which had previously been contested by industry, labor took the
position that it could obtain the financing of medical care through
the private sector by bargaining. This produced the great growth
in the United States of private health insurance. Prior to World
War II only 10% of the population had any form of health insurance,
but by the early 1950's, a majority of the population had some form
of health insurance through the private sector. While local and
national government had taken responsibility for some special
categories of risk in the population, nothing resembling general health
insurance was prevalent until the Blue Cross voluntary initiative
during the great depression of the 1930's. This had both the elements
of a consumer and producer cooperative. An occupational group,
schoolteachers, joined together and asked for care on a prepaid basis
from a hospital for the members of the group. Soon the hospitals
joined together and offered their services to groups on this basis.
Later in the 1940's surgeons formed similar producer cooperatives
for in-hospital procedures which became known as Blue Shield
Plans. Following these initiatives and the common acknowledgement of some employer obligation for these payments as a fringe
benefit, the large life and casualty insurance companies became active
in the field. It was voluntary, competitive free enterprise, typically
American.

Private health insurance had both its successes and its failures.
An analysis of this would require a lengthy discourse. However to
summarize very briefly, the eventuality after 25 years was that
the working population in general had coverage of its major in-
hospital expenses but not its ambulatory care. This put great emphasis
on acute hospital care. Those needy elements of society who had
either retired from work or who did not work regularly, or who
were self-employed, were left without health insurance and, because
of their need, found an actuarial barrier by experience rating to
obtaining it. These discrepancies in the midst of a progressively
affluent society proved to be intolerable to many, but change was
once again resisted by the medical profession.

A proposal to provide hospitalization to retired persons under the
Social Security Administration produced an elaborate and bitter

controversy that occupied the early 1960's. The controversy is very revealing as to the nature of the American value system (Harris, 1966). Finally, however, the passage in 1965 of modifications of the Social Security Act became known as Medicare and Medicaid. This is the second great watershed event in the history of health policy and compares with the Flexner Report in its degree of impact on the subsequent course of events. No single policy was embodied in these modifications of the Social Security Law, but a number of different policies were undertaken simultaneously. The Act is complex and cannot be represented to be otherwise. However, as an attempt to placate the medical profession, the very first section of the Act states firmly that no intent was present to change the nature of medical practice or its organization. Multiple differing philosophies of health financing were incorporated simultaneously. For hospitalization it became an inherent right for having worked under the Social Security system, but for professional services of physicians and surgeons, it became a voluntary contributory plan; and those not yet retired but who were in need became subject to an income test in a fiscal responsibility shared between the federal government and that of the states in such a manner that none of the 50 state jurisdictions have identical provisions for either eligibility or benefits. This has often been called a 'three-layer cake' but fundamentally represents intricate political compromise due to an inability to arrive at any general overall health policy.

Rapid changes in the costs of medical care and its regulation promptly ensued. Obviously the cost overruns which were in the billions of dollars and rapidly escalating were the primary consideration. This produced a profound dilemma for in part it competed with all other forms of federal spending.

Hasty attempts were also made through federal regulations to control the spending. From the official 'Conditions of Participation' through the 'Methods of Reimbursement', rigidity was placed in the system to the discomfiture of providers. The institutional health establishment was beset by turmoil, and the Administration and the Congress sought both explanations and scapegoats. Mr. Nixon, running for election in the fall of 1968, had proclaimed repeatedly that the United States had 'the best health care in the world'. He was inaugurated in January of 1969. By July 1969 his public pronouncements had completely reversed and he made his famous declaration of a 'health crisis', imputing that medical care must be reorganized or 'chaos would ensue'. Immediately a wide search was undertaken by the federal bureaucracy as to what alternative options were available in medical care. More than forty were explored.

An apparent partial solution to the health care problems besetting the Administration was felt to be embodied in the President's health message of 1971, in which he outlined the rationale for what was called the 'HMO' Policy. It is interesting that the acronym was said by the President before the name 'Health Maintenance Organization' was stated in full. The euphemistic character of the name apparently seems less a problem with its abbreviation, and so the latter has come into use almost independent of the words' meaning.

The antecedents of this form of organization date back forty years in America as 'Prepaid Group Practice' of which the Kaiser Medical Program has been the foremost example. The intent of the Administration, however, was to expand the concept to encompass a wider definition.

As this policy has developed a minimal definition has become necessary. An HMO is 1) an organized system in a geographical area, having responsibility for medical care for all its members; 2) provides a comprehensive set of basic benefits; 3) has voluntary enrollment, a continuous test of consumer satisfaction, and 4) is financed by a fixed periodic prepayment. This definition is designed to encompass both Prepaid Group Practice and Foundations for Medical Care, these being termed the centralized and decentralized forms of HMO. At the present time the overwhelming majority of members served by HMOs in the United States are served by Prepaid Group Practice. While Foundations for Medical Care have sprung up in many areas in the United States within the last four years, only a very small number of people are as yet being served by such organizations on a risk-taking basis which qualifies them as an HMO. The Foundations for Medical Care in many areas has limited its function to 'peer review' for appropriateness of services rendered (Steinwald, 1971). In a few areas it has assumed fixed payment risk for Medicaid populations. Prepaid Group Practice, of course, implies the physicians form a group and function as such in a common facility. In the 'Foundations for Medical Care' form the physicians practice in individual or small group offices being paid as individuals on a fee-for-service basis. The commonality is that of organizing to serve a voluntarily enrolled population for comprehensive services on a predetermined payment regardless of use of services. The HMO must be at actuarial risk or it is not an HMO.

Quite naturally as this was to be the Administration policy, a series of attempts were made over the next three years to legislatively implement it. Finally on December 30, 1973 an Act (P.L. 93-222) was signed into law to aid in the development of such organizations. Although it is an imperfect law it is a milestone of health policy formulation.

There were some obvious motivations for this approach. First, the prepaid group practice organizations had shown that they were cost saving. Such savings were generally estimated to be between 20 and 30 percent and were most clearly attributable to reduced hospitalization for the population served. The Foundations for Medical Care form had also begun to show significant reduction in hospital use. Obviously, to the Administration faced with huge cost overruns for Federal Medicare and Medicaid programs, a system that showed cost saving was an appealing alternative if, as had long been shown, the quality of care was at least equal. However, the appeal to the Administration and Congress went beyond this obvious cost awareness. The HMO was a competing, voluntary system, a reiteration of choice in a free market. It matched the avowed free enterprise policy. And perhaps more subtly, but nevertheless strongly, the concept of contracting the responsibility for the medical care of a voluntarily enrolled population also had appeal. Negotiation and contracting with an organization provides a method of control almost totally lacking in dealing with a myriad of individual practitioners paid fee for service, with only fragmented responsibility for patients, and none for populations. Government was on familiar ground in contracting with strong organizations that would deliver a product of desired specification for a firm price. Unorganized individual professional entrepreneurs, each of whom had only partial responsibility for a patient in his special field of practice, were beyond usual government management. The conventional form left the inherent dilemma of who was to take overall organized responsibility for defined populations.

Concomitant with this HMO activity, a new element had been injected into the national debate on health. In November 1968, the late Mr. Walter Reuther, the leader of the United Auto Workers Union, made a dramatic speech in which there was a call for national health insurance as an answer to the problems that the President was to admit the following summer (Reuther, 1969). Within the ensuing year a positive epidemic of proposals had occurred for national health insurance, coming from all parts of the establishment—from the American Medical Association, American Hospital Association, from Labor Unions, from the Administration and the various committees involved with health legislation of the Congress. Of more than twenty proposals, none called for a national health service. But despite the plethora of proposals, no legislation was enacted, and now after five years, none has been. Another concomitant reaction to the proclaimed health crisis was a further reorganization of the Department of Health, Education, and Welfare. The health functions were now once more relabled and again new civil servants were placed in high positions. The Administration's general theory was that the health sector had become so expensive it needed better management to reduce spending, and individuals distinguished in the general discipline of management, without regard necessarily to their experience in health, were made directors of large agencies. This lack of continuity of effort further thwarted production of consistent policy at a critical time.

The Congress, however, continued to respond with categorical approaches. For example, it favored cancer research and reacted with a 'Conquest of Cancer Program' costing half a billion dollars a year. It responded to care for end-stage renal disease with a dialysis and transplant program to which all are entitled. It made mandatory the assessment of the health status of disadvantaged children under Title 19 of the Social Security Act. It enacted the review of the quality of medical care under the Professional Standards Review Organizations (PSROs), projecting upon the profession a unique set of controls that exist in no other country. But there is no overall health policy. There is an ever increasing desire to control and regulate, and one sees medicine moving gradually toward the status of a public utility. This is a form in the United States in which historically those being regulated usually capture the regulatory agency (Havighurst, 1974).

This gradual forcing of the providers of health services in the United States into a controlled, regulated public utility model has been the reaction of government to the responsibility of financing care for but the 10% of the people who are over 65 years of age and the 10% of people who are otherwise economically disadvantaged in American society. In other words, to provide the health care financing for 20% of the people, perhaps the most needy 20%, all of health services are being pushed into a form of public control that provides a constant constraint upon the providers. The medical profession in the United States quite clearly does not wish to participate in such controls. It asserts and reasserts the traditional American values of individual competition and free enterprise. The paradox is that the government also continually asserts these values, stating the great value of pluralism in our society, but at the same time produces the regulations and controls that inhibit the free interactions said to be desired. An open question in the minds of those concerned with national health insurance is that when 100% of the people, rather than the present 20%, become entitled by national health insurance which must then be regulated by government, how will the values so firmly held, of competition and pluralism, be possible?

In the future, when National Health Insurance has been established for a few years, and the backlog of deficits of medical service have been met, and there is a relatively constant level of operations, one would expect that the ability to expand the resource allocation to health services at an even greater rate would come into formidable conflict with other societal priorities. Health spending in the United States is between 7½ and 8 percent of the Gross National Product, and the percentage has been rising. This amounts to $104 billion in the 1974 fiscal year. It is felt that it will continue to rise as the backlog of needs is made up, but then will plateau into a relatively constant relationship with the growth of the Gross National Product. As this occurs, with all citizens entitled to a comprehensive set of health services through national health insurance, the arguments about equity of different segments of the population in access to health services of comparable quality and in comparable facilities will force a major reordering of priorities and a rethinking of the values of medical service.

Most experts would agree that medical care services are but one ingredient in the health of a population and such factors as education, employment, housing, nutrition, sanitation, and other environmental factors make equally large contributions. But as this becomes generally apparent, it will not lessen the desire for the caring or curing functions of medicine but will force the reordering of the priorities of resource allocation. As these interactions occur it is predictable that a national health policy will be forged in which expression is given to these conflicting factors and a more general overall plan elaborated. This policy it would seem must be consonant with the overall expressed set of cultural values and attitudes in regard to competition, freedom, and pluralism. One can discern some, but by no means all, of the outcomes of this process. It is possible that it will fundamentally reorganize the structure of health services in the United States.

The current controversy indicates wide agreement in one area in that there must be pluralism. The canard of 'monolithic' has defeated some proposals before rational debate occurred. What is not so clear is whether the policy issue of pluralism must extend to financing mechanisms or whether only to the health services delivery mechanisms. The latter seems to be the more crucial attribute.

Is there a delivery system that within a finite resource allocation can produce a sense of equity, a sense of responsibility and consumer satisfaction? Long experience has told us that the present individual practitioner, individual hospital, patient-oriented, piecework payment system hasn't produced either equity or fiscal responsibility. There are probably many other ways, but it proves difficult to formulate many given all the other values of our society.

A relevant aspect of the HMO Policy is this element of voluntary choice and inherent competition. Section 1310 of the HMO Act of

1973 calls for mandatory offering of this competing form wherever health benefits are offered by employers. Employer contribution, in whole or in part, is the present dominant form of financing health benefits in America, so such a requirement is intended to widely invoke the free market mechanism. The HMO form is not perfect and need not be perfect, but it is a viable competitor. It has inherently most of the qualities necessary to meet the hypothesized conditions of the period after National Health Insurance is enacted.

The HMO format, although existing for the past forty years, never received federal interest until federal responsibility for payment for medical services in Medicare and Medicaid was assumed. Now, however, the potential of cost saving by placing the delivery system at risk financially has appeal to the federal budget makers. Obviously one of the few forms of organization that has already experienced this actuarial risk on scale has been the Prepaid Group Practice-Health Maintenance Organization. Here there is a capitated budget, a population for which to be responsible, and the continual delicate test of voluntary membership in a multiple-choice market. Here morbidity (in contrast to fee-for-service) is not an asset to the providers but a liability. In such a setting the urge is to do only what is appropriate, to do it at the earliest effective opportunity, and to do it as efficiently as possible. The experience of long years of operations at large-scale and at multiple sites under different leaders has produced a reasonable, but by no means rigid, consensus on the specifications. The form is derived from the function.

Because of the assumption of risk for enrolled membership at a prospectively budgeted rate, and because of the internal controls (although differing) that each has, and because consumers perceive them as offering fundamentally different choices, the Foundations for Medical Care and Prepaid Group Practice forms of HMO appear to be models adaptable to the period after National Health Insurance. One could predict over a period of years a strong evolution of even the majority of medical practice to these two differently perceived, cost-controlling mechanisms. Each has an effect on efficiency. Although the more organized Prepaid Group Practice form has a greater effect, that of the Foundations for Medical Care will be considerable. Health policy will strongly favor these cost-controlling forms due to economic pressure, particularly as it still leaves a choice of system of medical care.

After universal entitlement is enacted, health services will need some form of politically responsive governance to assure reasonable equity within a finite resource allocation. This cannot be done by health professionals alone. Nor can it be done effectively by federal administrators alone. Some form of Regional Health Authority becomes a political necessity for response to consumer pressure. A long history of attempts at significant regionalization efforts has met with only marginal success. The Hill-Burton legislation for hospital construction of 1945 called for regional planning, and this planning met with less than spectacular success. The Regional Medical Program Act of 1965 attempted a regional technical recourse rationalization. Comprehensive Health Planning legislation has been striving for meaningful local institutional integration (through '314 B' agencies) for eight years. The recent PSRO legislation has created 203 new 'local areas' for a specific medical quality control function. Further strong indication of the attempt to rationalize health services on a regional basis comes from the release of the final policies for endstage renal disease under Medicare. On April 17, 1974, Assistant Secretary of Health, Education and Welfare, Charles Edwards, M.D., stated that services would only be provided by 'networks of facilities and services on a regional basis to match need'. He further generalized—

If we are going to be able to assure quality health care, not just for kidney disease patients but for everyone, and if we are going to make such care available universally at a cost that the American people can afford, then we are going to have to develop the kind of rational balanced systems such as the one we have put together for the kidney program.

With the aggregate cost of health services in this country now at $100 billion a year and climbing, with economic controls about to be taken off the health care industry, and with National Health Insurance plainly on the horizon—we have to devise sound, rational, and efficient systems of health care financing and delivery. I think the kidney disease program is an example of what can be accomplished in the public-private sector if we have the will. And there can be no question that we have the need.

It seems quite reasonable that if there were one or more HMOs in such a regional authority that would enroll members voluntarily and obligate itself to provide ready access to the mandated, comprehensive services for a predetermined annual payment, the health funding source would be most eager to cooperate and contract the obligation. There is every indication that contracting of responsibility is desired. This process has already occurred as a form of state budgetary (and hence tax) control in California for the Medicaid population. It is spreading to New York, Maryland, and other states as a way to control Medicaid costs. Performance is to be audited as a matter of contract.

If there were a voluntary choice of HMOs of different types, Foundations for Medical Care or Prepaid Group Practice, or of HMO and non-HMO, there would be in time a clear vote as to which system produced consumer satisfaction. Instead of a public utility type institution on a budget having a program substantially motivated by its ability to expand its allocated budget, the voluntary HMO would have the continuous test of the market by being able to grow only if it produced consumer satisfaction.

In summary, we see ourselves in the midst of a transition as to health policy and the organization of health services. Such policy largely reflects the attitudes, culture, and customs of the society interacting with a traditional profession. Our society prides itself on free enterprise, the independence of the individual, and free institutions. Medical care has well reflected this.

Few seem to see that our classic mode of financing medical services by fees and charges has shaped what are the present characteristics of the profession and health institutions.

But just as the present method of paying shapes the present system so will the financing method of any national health insurance affect the delivery system. Public finite resource allocation to the health sector, publicly regulated and publicly debated, will force a discussion of priorities and hence develop policy.

The policy will embody the central cultural values that are characteristic of the society. There may or may not be pluralism of the funding sources for health. This is not the central issue with the public, although for obvious reasons it is of paramount importance to the private insurance industry. Much of the medical profession is concerned only that unified funding might cause unified control.

However, one can be reasonably certain that the finite resource allocation under public review will promote a choice of competing systems of health services. It appears to be the American way.

Bibliography

1. American Medical News (August 5, 1974), p. 8. Chicago: American Medical Association.
2. Carnegie Commission on Higher Education (1970). *Higher Education and the Nation's Health, Policies for Medical and Dental Education*, p. 25. New York: McGraw-Hill.
3. Committee on the Costs of Medical Care (adopted October 31, 1932). *Medical Care for the American People, the Final Report*. Chicago: The University of Chicago Press, reprinted by the United States Department of Health, Education, and Welfare (1970).
4. Harris, R. (1966) in *A Sacred Trust*, p. 218. New York: New American Library.
5. *Regulating Health Facilities Construction* (1974), ed. Havighurst, C. C. Washington, D.C.: American Enterprise Institute for Public Policy Research.

6. Reuther, W. P. (1969). *The Health Care Crisis: Where Do we go from Here?*, The Eighth Bronfman Lecture. Detroit: American Public Health Association.
7. Steinwald, C. (1971). Blue Cross Reports, Research Series 7. Chicago: Blue Cross Association.
8. United States Congress (1971). House Document No. 49, 92nd Congress. Washington, D.C.: United States Government Printing Office.
9. United States Department of Health, Education, and Welfare, Public Health Service (1974). Remarks by Edwards, C. C. Washington, D.C.: United States Government Printing Office.

Chapter 16

MEDICAL CARE IN NORWAY

C. F. BORCHGREVINK
Institut for Almenmedisin, Oslo, Norway

NORWAY HAS for many years been a very pleasant, quiet and peaceful place to live. It is fairly large, 320.000 km² = 125.000 square miles with a population of 4 mill., giving a density of 12 people pr. km², i.e. the less densely populated country on the European Continent. The coastline including the fjords is about 21.000 km, and from north to south is equivalent from Oxford to North Africa. Norway stretches surprisingly far up towards the North Pole where the sun is never to be seen for several months during winter. Many people feel that God never intended Norway to be inhabited, but thanks to the Gulf-stream it *is* possible. The political situation has been stable, with surprisingly small differences between the major parties in socio-political problems.

Norway is not a rich country using the western standard, but with the oil in the North Sea we shall for a short while be wealthy with *all* the problems that involves.

With this background let us look at our health care system and its influence upon education, hospital-service and the provision of medical care in the community. Discussing the problems of personnel, I shall concentrate upon the role of the doctor, leaving out nurses, social workers, district nurses, physiotherapists and so on. Not because they play a less important role in the health system, but because it seemed to me that the program of this symposium was directed towards the work and role of the doctor. Of course doctors are important, but so are the other health personnel, and one may well argue that if you were to have only one of the groups of health personnel, you would do very well with district nurses.

In 1911 a State-operated, non-profit insurance program was organized, which was compulsory for the lower income groups. This program had gradually been enlarged until the membership was made compulsory for everybody in 1956. More services have been added, and in 1967 the National Insurance was established as an integrated and coordinated social insurance system, which covers medical care and pensions. Doctors in practice work on a fee-for-service basis, and the patients pay part of their fee: about 40% at the first visit, and less for the second visit and nothing for the third and later visits. Hospitals are publicly owned: hospital doctors work full time on salary, but are in addition allowed 5-6 hours private practice a week. Hospital treatment is free. Essential drugs used outside hospitals are paid for by the program, less important ones and drugs you will only need for a short time are paid by the patient. Surprisingly, dental care is generally not included. Considering the *need* for dental care service, and considering the great difference in the use of this service between the social classes, it must be considered one of the black spots in our health care that dental service is not free to everyone.

The expenses have increased rapidly. Between 1961 and 1971 public expenses for health and welfare increased from 10,9 to 17,4% of the gross national product, and the average increase in public expenses for health and welfare went up from 13% for 1961–66 to 22% for 1971–72 (Hjort 1973).

In the early years of this century the growth of medical knowledge and specialization began to require larger administrative units (the 20 counties) especially for hospitals. Each county has a medical team, which is responsible for supervision and planning of health care in the county. Its special duty is to develop a complete health plan for the county, including a hospital program. The system is managed centrally by a Directorate of Health, under the Department of Social Affairs.

Outside hospital the patients may in principle see the general practitioner they want, and may freely circulate between several practitioners if they so wish. However, in large part of the country the population has but one doctor, the district medical officer, and the free choice of doctor is in fact an illusion.

In order to see a specialist, except for pediatricians, you will have to be referred by a general practitioner. This means referred and not transferred. The administration, especially in the bigger towns, wants to change this, because they feel the system would be easier to handle if the patient could visit a specialist directly. They have introduced the system in Oslo and Bergen, but I hope we shall be able to go back to the older referral system, as I definitely believe that patients are best served by their family doctor, a generalist, who, when necessary should refer him to the specialist, and guide the patient through the medical jungle we have created. It is often difficult for the patient himself to select the proper specialist when symptoms are vague.

To meet the growing expectation for better medical care, Norway has about 6.700 doctors, one doctor pr. 580 inhabitants. This does not sound too bad, but the situation in many places is quite difficult because of the maldistribution.

Particularly the specialists want to work in towns or densely populated areas. The 1600 general practitioners are fairly evenly distributed, but considering the long distances in the Northern Norway, and partly in the West, the people in these areas could do with some more general practitioners. The home-visit may easily take as much as a day, since air-service is not well developed.

Of the 1600 general practitioners, 450 are district medical officers, appointed by the government, with a fixed salary for their public health duties. In addition they do general practice on the usual fee-for-service basis, which contributes largely to their income. There are for the moment practically no vacancies in these jobs, which in spite of long working days, often isolated places, are very attractive, especially among young doctors. Unfortunately the wives often see it in the different light, and for this reason there is considerable turnover in the jobs.

In spite of the seemingly satisfactory patient/doctor ratio, most of the doctors work long hours, on an average 55 hours pr. week. The district medical officer in the North has 70 hours pr. week or more, time for studying *not* included.

Because of these many hours, the doctors' income is highly satisfactory, and some doctors have such a high income that it has drawn a negative attention from the government, and to a lesser extent from the public. However, based on a normal working week of 40 hours, one cannot say that the doctors are overpaid. The average income is about £10.000, 2% earn more than £20.000, and 8% less than £7.500.

Norway has 200 somatic hospitals including 65 small cottage hospitals, average 20 beds, run by the district medical officer. There are 22.000 somatic beds giving 5,5 somatic beds pr. 1000 population. There is quite a variation between the counties, 7,4 in Oslo to 2,8 in a county in western Norway.

In addition there are 3,5 psychiatric beds pr. 1000 population which may be more than enough, as more and more of the psychiatric treatment takes place in outpatient clinics or at home.

Norway has 18.000 beds in nursing-homes, and there are plans to increase this number by 2000 a year until 28.000.

Some new hospitals are planned, and a few must be rebuilt or remodelled, but on the whole it is felt that the number of hospital beds are sufficient if they could be used more effectively. If old and disabled persons who need to be looked after, but do not need intensive medical care and who at the present occupy as much as 30% of the beds in the medical ward, could be moved to nursing-homes, where they probably would be better off anyway, we may already have the adequate number of somatic beds.

The Parliament will probably next year be debating a bill for future expansion of our hospital service, based on the need and the wishes, of the 20 counties. According to this plan we shall have 4 major hospitals (regional hospitals), at least one large central hospital in each county with most specialities, and decentralized smaller hospitals in the community, including surgery, medicine, and x-ray departments. In addition we shall probably still need smaller cottage hospitals run by the district medical officer because of the long distances in part of the country.

Together with this debate in Parliament, there will be a corresponding debate on the health-service in the community. So far the responsibility of the government has been to appoint 450 district medical officers scattered all over the country. The further development of medical practice outside hospitals, both specialist and general practice, has been left partly to the private initiative of doctors and partly to the Norwegian Medical Association. In wide circles this is no longer satisfactory, and most likely the responsibility for planning community health service, both preventive, curative and rehabilitation, will be delegated to the counties, and integrated with the plans for hospital service.

Norway has three medical schools, the fourth opened in 1975, but only for the clinical medicine. The medical curriculum lasts 6 years. In our two larger medical schools the curriculum is traditional with strict separation between clinical and preclinical medicine. In the Tromsø medical school far North, which opened in 1973, there will be an integration both between preclinical and clinical medicine, and between university and society. The students will for instance work for 4 months outside the teaching hospital in smaller hospitals in Northern Norway, and in addition they will spend 2 months with a district medical officer.

325 students enter medical school each year, and there are less than 10% dropouts during the study. In addition between 100 and 150 students go abroad to study medicine to the eternal shame of Norwegian medicine, because we do not have the facilities to educate them at home.

The goal of the study is to produce a general practitioner who is ready to take responsibility for independent work anywhere in the country. Strangely enough the planners of the curriculum have never really tried to analyse what the general practitioner should do in the future, and what he needs of knowledge and skills to carry out his duty. According to the Norwegian sociologists Løchen (1971) many general practitioners are overqualified in certain aspects of medicine and highly under-qualified in others. This leads to frustration and may be one of the major reasons while for some time general practitioners have left their profession and looked for jobs in hospitals.

We have carried out an analysis of the workload of the general practitioner. It turned out that about one out of five patients has complaints from the skeleton/muscle system, and almost the same number visits the doctor because of minor psychiatric problems. The two groups of diseases are also the most important ones in relation to sick leave and disability. Considering their importance, it is surprising that the two fields are poorly covered in the curriculum. This brings me to the following important problem. There are at least two ways in looking at the relation between education and health care. Either you define the need for health care, and plan the education accordingly (the ideal way), or, and this is what happens, you educate doctors in a certain way, usually according to tradition, and you get the health care they are educated for, which in Norway so far has produced an excellent hospital medicine and service and hospitalminded doctors, but has so far been less satisfactory to the delivery of community health. I would think it is correct to say that the most important way to influence the health care system is not necessarily through bills or politicians, but through the medical curriculum, because, as I said, the doctors to a large extent will carry out the jobs they are trained for more or less regardless of the intention of the Department of Social Affairs.

Some years ago I heard that Royal College in this country was not interested in politics, only in education. Indeed a remarkable statement.

These thoughts are, of course, neither original nor particularly brilliant, still they have been slow in penetrating to the University and Health-authorities. At the Medical Faculty in Oslo a committee has now been appointed to plan a new curriculum where community medicine will be given a major role. Furthermore our four medical schools have recently established departments of general practice in addition to departments of social medicine.

By changing the rules and regulations for admitting students to the medical faculty, with more emphasis on motivation and less on performance in school, we hope that the next generation of doctors will be more patient and community oriented.

To encourage doctors to go into general practice a postgraduate and continuous education program for general practitioners have been adopted. General practice is still not a speciality, but the doctor who takes the recommended (not compulsory) education will be some kind of a specialist. You need about five years to become a specialist in most subjects, a general practitioner will have three year postgraduate training (two of which in general practice) and three hundred hours of courses, tailored for general practice. As continuous education he must have two weeks courses every year and three months hospital service every five years.

Conclusion: Our medical care system is of course not perfect, but it must be considered fairly satisfactory. It gives within geographic limitations the same service to every citizen, regardless of income and social class. The fee-for-service system encourages the doctor to work hard and since there probably always will be a shortage of doctors, this may be an advantage. However, having a different system of payment for the various group of health-personnel, as the others are on a fixed salary, is a disadvantage, and makes it more difficult to obtain an integrated health service. The system has not successfully coped with the problem of even distribution of doctors throughout the country, in particular not for specialists. A 100% ideal distribution can of course never be obtained, but we ought to do better than we have.

Our system encourages curative medicine at the expense of preventive medicine. It will always be difficult to make the right priority between curative and preventive medicine, but in my mind we shall have to allocate more of our resources to the field of preventive medicine. The whole problem of prevention is getting more and more complicated. Previously prevention of diseases was a medical problem, which medicine more or less has solved with regard to infectious diseases. Today prevention is just as much a political problem. To a large extent we have the knowledge to prevent or at least reduce cardiovascular diseases, lung cancer, traffic accidents, but for many reasons, some of which are good and valid, the government is not willing to take the necessary steps.

On the whole our medical system has been little criticized even if there are political trends that want to abolish the fee-for-service system and have all doctors on fixed salary. There is no wish neither from Directorate of Health nor from the Medical Faculty drastically to change the medical education. Barefoot doctors do not seem to be the answer to our problems.

If one accepts that Norway has a reasonable medical care system of today, the future may be more of a problem. The medical knowledge does increase, the expectations to medical care increases correspondingly, or even more rapidly, but resources both in manpower and money do not keep pace with the rising expectations and increased knowledge. Consequently the gap between what we have the knowledge to do, and what we in practice are able to do becomes wider and wider. I think we shall have to accept that we must reduce our level of ambition.

Life expectancy for women is 77 and men 71 years, and even if

we still may add some more years by successfully fighting, e.g.
coronary heart disease, a lot can be said that at this stage it is
equally important to improve the *quality* of life as it is to prolong
life. As Cochrane (1972) said 'Cure is the enemy of care'. This is
becoming an issue in Norway where many of us feel that the dying
patient is not getting the care he deserves, probably simply because
he cannot be cured. Fortunately the various aspects of terminal care
are more frequently discussed these days.

It is obvious that in the future the demand for health services
will be much greater than the available resources. In order to arrive
at sensible priorities in such a situation we will need more information. How can we best spend our millions? Where and how
can the personnel be of most and best use? Is home-care cheaper
than hospital-care? What is best: To centralize or decentralize
health-service? Or rather: How far should decentralization go?
Such questions will always be difficult to answer, may be impossible,
but an independent institution for health economy or better health
priorities may perhaps provide us with solutions in the future, when
we will be able more successfully to analyse such problems and to
evaluate the data which can be provided.

References

Cochrane, A. L. (1972): *Effectiveness and efficiency*, pp 92, The Nuffield
  Provincial Hospitals Trust, Burgess & Son (Abingdon) Ltd., London.
Hjort, P. F. (1973) *Medical education, care, and research in Norway*, Ciba
  Foundation Symposium 21, pp 153-165, Elsevier, Amsterdam.
Løchen, Y. (1971): *Behandlingssamfunnet*, pp 40-103, Gyldendal Norsk
  Forlag, Oslo.

Chapter 17

MEDICAL CARE IN DENMARK

G. ALMIND
Holbaek, Denmark

DENMARK HAS had a kind of health insurance as in many other European countries, until a few years ago. Then we changed to a system quite near to the British National Health System. It means that all costs to medical care, except for a part of medicine and a few exceptions of doctors' salaries, are paid by the taxes.

The primary medical care is based on general practitioners, which are covering the country fairly uniform with 1 : 2,400 inhabitants. We are feeling, that we have a lack of GPs on the other hand, for the time being we are educating too many students and as soon as they have passed the postgraduate training, there will become too many doctors in Denmark. A few have already started to emigrate to New Zealand and USA.

The people can normally contact their own GP in the daytime, and if necessary get a home-visit. During the night they can get a doctor and outside Copenhagen often their own or one from the group. 20% of GPs are now working in groups of more than 2 doctors, and the numbers are increasing.

The family doctors are paid in a mixed per head and fee for service salary. As a relic from the insurance-time the population is divided into two groups: 1. consisting of 85%, paying nothing to the GP, but have to use the same GP and need a letter of permission to specialists from their doctor. The doctor can be changed once a year, but only 1% of the population is using that right. 2. consisting of 15% with the highest incomes, are free to change doctors as often as they want and go directly to the specialist. Nevertheless the main part is using their family doctor. This group has to pay the doctor themselves, but a part (approximately 3/5) will be reimbursed.

Next year this will be changed in the way that all people can choose whether they want to join group 1 or 2, with the possibility to change once a year.

Specialists and hospitalization is available after a fairly reasonable waiting-time, i.e. from a cut from up to one year for hernias and various other disorders. I do not know if the waiting time is necessary, but I think it has nothing to do with the number of hospital beds. It is a normal component of an official system, because it is giving a steady intake to the hospitals and it is one of the ways the hospitals are pressing for new appropriations.

The main part of the hospitals are new, mostly built during the last 15 years or totally renewed. In the same time we have got many new nursing homes specially for people needing care all day and night, and a number of local medical centres have been erected, and paid for by the doctors. The institutions are well-built and equipped, many people feel, that they are too good.

In spite of the many good things you can say about the system, a part of the population is unsatisfied and there are an increasing number of complaints. During the late summer we have had several broad- and tele-casts dealing with the matter and the doctors have not been lucky each time they were interviewed. The complaints concern very often small matters and are easy and correctly rejected, but their origin must be found in problems as lack of engagement or interest from the doctors, cool climate in the institutions among them the new local health centres, and the patient and his relatives feeling of being dissatisfied.

Increasing Expenses

The increasing expenses to the health budget are known in all countries, in Denmark it has been going up from 3.9 to 5.7% of the GNP during the last 15 years, and it is now clear, that none of the political parties will allow further increases. In another way you can imagine: 4% of people in the age of 18–66 are taking care of 8% of temporary ill or pensioners in the same ages. It means that 12% are nonproductive.

The new social system

The most important event for the Danish GP's has been the new social reform, which gradually is being introduced during the years by several laws. The Danish Medical Association (including all physicians) was not taking part in the committee-work in the begining, but since it has appeared that it will include considerable changes, particularly the job of the GPs the DMA has joined the further work.

The idea is that all social problems shall be treated in a one-string system, consisting of social centres in the municipalities (min. population of 5,000). Problems needing specialists are solved in the social centre of the county (1/4–1/2 million) and the planning education and principles are dealt with at state level (5 million).

In the municipalities only one person or a little group of persons take care of the family, and one can present all social problems here (housing, rehabilitation, economy, child welfare etc). The group try to solve the total problem and not only a small part of it. All questions about pensions, admittance to nursing homes, special flats and day-centres for pensioners, payment of money for days lost through sickness, delivery or accidents, is gathered in this centre, and here the people decide who they want as the family doctor.

Everybody is still free to go directly to the GP and is doing so (the GPs are in contact with 1.6% of the population each day), but it has been recognised, as you can imagine, that people frequently using the social centre are well-known by the doctor, that many problems presented in the social centre have a medical solution for a bigger or smaller part, and the other way round.

Thus there are an increasing number of contacts between the health and social centre. The physicians closest co-worker, except for nurses and secretaries working in the health centre, as home nurses, health visitors and home visitors are placed in the social centre too. It seems peculiar, that we in general practice still are able to work as a partly liberal part of the system, with a partly fee-for-service payment, unlimited number of patients, self-financing and unrestricted right to decide about co-workers in the practice and technical equipment.

The social centre in the county takes care of adoptions, allocation of pensions, supervisors and specialists to the municipalities, social workers to the hospitals, special out-patient clinics for family-problems, addicts, day-and-night homes for alcoholics, children, pensioners, etc.

In the 'health string' all hospitals (with very few exceptions) are placed and owned on county level. The social functions on county level requires a lot of doctors, normally coming from the specialists in the hospitals.

Until now the system has been a considerable step forward and the idea of 'one gate' to the social system and the decisions made known to the patient—in the future, with the patient I hope—has been accepted by people as a positive thing. On the other hand one must realize, that the increasing number of contacts between the physicians and the social centre have not been followed by a change in the number of contacts with the patient, that the power of the combination doctor-social centre is enormous, and the patient has no choice but following their decisions. The professional secrecy is giving problems too.

Two other strings are of importance for the future work of the doctors, the educational and the occupational. We have had for many years school doctors, but have just started to create an occupational health system, mainly based on general practitioners.

Health Education

In Denmark too we have realised that the necessary stop in the increase of health-expenses must lead to other and cheaper possibilities. One of the ways is to develop the traditional preventive medicine in the direction of health education. Since the problem now in many ways is the same all over the world, it must be possible to profit by international experiences.

It is very difficult to say how this shall be done, but a good deal of research has already been done in our ranks and we will be able to profit from advertising and political publicity. But further experience must be gained and the results published and studied. The school for children is an institution that most countries possess, often under continuous renewal and, first of all, the health education must be placed here and perhaps for a part already in the pre-school time, where preventive medicine has a traditional place. It should be based on sincere acceptance of, and fair information about, the true conditions the children are living in, and will be living in : hard work, frequent change of work, stimulations such as drugs, tobacco and alcohol, pollution, venereal diseases, malnutrition, too little and mainly too much to eat, and still in many countries too many early pregnancies. Information about these problems, their origin, their influence of health, why the generation of their parents has created a world like this, and accepted many of the problems, will make it easier for the children to understand and take our advice, in order to learn to take care of their health.

Teachers, social workers and journalists must take their part, but the people in the health system, particularly the doctors, are important because of their scientific background and experience in health problems second to none.

The health system has developed in most countries without the help or interference of the patient directly. The influence of the patient through elected persons, i.e. elected local or central politicians are not acceptable, because the politicians are in a way questioned as to whether they are a genuine patient. They are looking upon the costs, etc. We need more collaboration with the patient, when we are going to plan future health systems.

Chapter 18

MEDICAL CARE IN SWEDEN

FRANZ R. BÁRÁNY
St. Erik's Hospital, Stockholm, Sweden

MEDICAL CARE in Sweden is paid for mainly out of local taxation. There are still a considerable number of private practitioners but at the hospitals, which are run by the county councils, private practice was completely abolished in 1970. Within the next two years the social democratic government intends to bring all private practice into the county service by an agreement like that made this year with the dental profession. A scale of fees for every type of consultation and treatment is being worked out; the patient pays a certain fraction of the cost to the doctor, who then gets the rest from the county council via the health insurance board.

These are the last steps in a development over about 40 years in which medical care in Sweden has been transformed from a loosely organized activity with much freedom and scope for private initiative, especially on the part of the doctors, to a fully organized and centralized social service. Obviously this has involved the establishment of a bureaucracy, and most of the power of decision-making has been transferred from the doctors to the administrators. Up to now the gains of this reorganization in my opinion have not been very great. But we must admit that significant imperfections also existed in the previous system, some of which have been eliminated as a matter of course along with the direct financial interest of the medical profession. For the patient this has been of limited value. Instead, the public has suffered obvious disadvantages from the dehumanization and alienation which is liable to attend all bureaucratic structures. When this affects people who are bodily, mentally, or socially handicapped, the difficulty of finding their way through the multitude of red tape is especially great. The cries for help from the sufferers have, at least until now, not reached into the planning offices of the top administrators. Their planning is built on statistical data, which have little to do with the situation of the sick individual. One of the main reasons for this is that the officials who are fit people trained to think on economic lines cannot or will not understand the great gap that exists between the anxiety of the person who suddenly notices symptoms of illness, and the final, often trifling diagnosis made by the doctor after investigations.

Available resources

Hospitals. In Table I (p. 190) the number of hospitals of different categories is shown. They serve our population of about 8 million people. The 70 basic hospitals all have departments for the 5 basic activities—internal medicine, surgery, long term care (including facilities for physical rehabilitation), radiology, and anesthesiology. Some of them carry on one or more further activities. The 24 county hospitals usually have between 15 and 20 spheres of activity. The 9 provincial hospitals, one for each of the 9 provinces of Sweden, have about 30. The catchment area of each of these provincial hospitals contains about a million people; for the county hospitals this figure is somewhat over 300,000, and for the basic hospitals somewhat over 100,000. The number of doctors employed in hospitals is about 6650; 3150 of these have higher qualifications or are specialists; the remaining 3500 are still under postgraduate training.

Non-hospital and out-patients care. This is of three types. The *out-patients departments* in hospitals cover about 50% of all consultations. *General practitioners* cover about 25% and *practising specialists* the remaining 25%. In the two last groups about half are private practitioners. These approximately 1000 doctors in private practice thus cover about 25% of the non-hospital care, or about as much as the publicly employed general practitioners and specialists.

The public health services in 1971 were composed of 550 single-doctor practices, 125 two-doctor practices, and 65 three- (or more) doctor practices. About 1000 doctors, and 100 locums, work in these public services. In addition, about 450 doctors are engaged exclusively on out-patient care at hospitals. The *greater* part of the out-patient services is undertaken by doctors for whom this work represents a smaller part of their duties.

Personnel. Table II (p. 191) shows in the first column the number of doctors in 1972. We will come back to the other columns later. Table III (p. 191) shows the number of trained nurses.

Cost. Table IV (p. 191) shows the annual costs for medical care in the last years. The sum total of 8400 millions kronor implies that we pay just over 1000 kronor per head each year for our public medical services. To this we must add the benefits paid out in cash for sick-pensioning (a cost which I have not been able to ascertain); the cash benefits from national health insurance which in 1970 amounted to 2700 millions; and the cost for education of all personnel employed in medical care (again not ascertained). So, in fact, each person in Sweden pays probably nearly 2000 kronor, which is about 200 pounds, each year for medical care, medical education, and cash benefits including incapacity pensions.

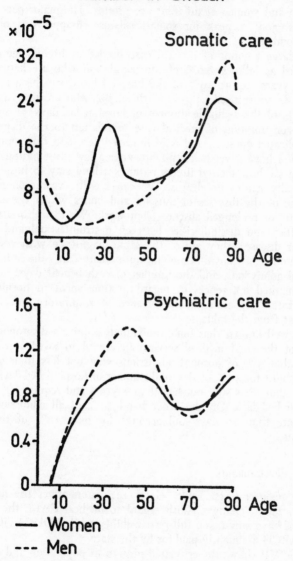

Fig. 1. Annual discharge rates from somatic hospital departments (1965–1968) and from psychiatric hospital departments (1968).

Consumption of medical care

Fig. 1 (p. 187) shows the number of discharges from Swedish hospitals for men and women at different age groups. The major part of the womens' 30-year peak for somatic disease disappears if obstetric care is omitted.

The large amount of medical care needed at higher age can be expressed as follows. 8.6% of the population who are between 65 and 74 years require 19% of the hospital bed-days; the 4.1% who are 75–84 years need 21%; and the 0.7% who are over 85 years need 9% of the available number of hospital bed-days.

The consumption of medical care in relation to the diagnosis is a complicated question and is of limited interest in this context. In Table V I have nevertheless put together a few illuminating figures. We can see how mental illness requires a long stay in hospital but statistically causes no deaths. We can see the vast economic importance of the diseases of muscles and bones which lies in their high rate of prolonged absence from work. We can also study the similarities and dissimilarities between gastrointestinal and cardiovascular disease: they are of the same magnitude with respect to the number of consultations in out-patient care, the number of hospital admissions, and the number of cash benefit days; but they show marked differences in regard to time spent in hospital and death rate. The economic importance of respiratory infections is apparent from the table.

It is well known that some individuals require a disproportionate share of the total medical service. In regard to Sweden it can be stated that 5% of hospital admissions stay not less than 90 days and account for 50% of the total number of hospital bed-days. 0.4% of the admissions stay not less than 2 years and require 20% of the hospital bed-days. On the other hand 50% of all admissions stay not more than 10 days and account for only 10% of the total available.

Future developments

Fundamental facts. Table VI (p. 192) summarizes the most important recent changes. With regard to medical CARE the county councils have now taken full responsibility while EDUCATION and RESEARCH are mainly paid for by the state.

Table VII shows the estimated growth in population and changes in age distribution until the end of the century. As can be seen the age-group 70–79 increases considerably both in absolute and relative terms until the end of the 1980's, after which it decreases.

The very highest age-groups, however, which require much care and nursing, continue to increase throughout the whole period.

For a long time there has been migration in Sweden from the country to towns and cities. Besides, statistically it appears that the whole growth in the population has taken place in urbanized areas. Around 1930 about half the total population of 6 millions lived in sparsely populated areas. In 1970 less than 20% of the 8.1 millions lived in these areas. The importance of this continuous migration for the planning of medical care is of course diminished by improved transport facilities.

Public demands. The demand for higher standards in medical care follows more or less automatically the rise in the standard of living. If we are not too pessimistic with respect to this rise, one can forsee several lines along which this demand will express itself.

1. More differentiated and highly qualified medical service within easy reach. A study in Göteborg showed that this is what the public wants: even for episodic acute disease people want to consult a highly qualified doctor.
2. Less institutionalized care. More help for the old, disabled, and handicapped to remain in their normal surroundings. This also lays claims on the medical organization for better service within easy reach.
3. Strengthened industrial health service. Strong demands for this are expressed by the trade unions. These demands also include efforts for the prevention of injuries caused by work in factories. This again calls for an increase in medical, technical, and behaviouristic competence.
4. Medical progress. Perhaps it is wrong to speak of public demand in this context, but what is being planned or introduced in Sweden now, and what one would like the public to take an interest in and help get money for, are the following preventive measures:

(a) a greatly increased vaccination program covering measles, german measles, and other virus diseases, possibly in the near future also some types of malignant disease;
(b) more—and more effective—advisory boards for problem families and also for family planning;
(c) increased facilities for preventive health checks, which are directed towards certain groups of people who are particularly exposed to certain industrial diseases and hazards;
(d) special facilities for the detection and care of patients with high blood pressure;

(e) attempts to change our habits in regard to diet, smoking, and taking physical exercise;

(f) augmentation of the facilities for genetic and metabolic diagnostics aiming at the identification during pregnancy of such irregularities which may damage the embryo;

(g) intensified and improved preventive pharmacotherapy, like e.g. lithium prophylaxis in mano-depressive disease.

Future resources. In Table II (p. 191) I have estimated the number of available doctors in the near future. A reasonable balance will be reached in 1985 between the number of highly qualified doctors and those still under training, which should make life easier for the former group than it is now.

The number of nurses, Table III, is believed to be sufficient throughout. Few new hospitals will be needed, it is supposed, but a considerable number of new health centers and nursing-homes for the old and disabled will be required. The economic growth in our country is estimated at about 4% per annum. This constitutes a framework within which public expenditure must remain to avoid endangering the social economic balance. A yearly expansion of 4% for medical services cannot be achieved without increased taxation because of the labour-intensive nature of medical care.

REFERENCES

Riksförsäkringsverket: Statistisk Rapport Nr 1974:1, Stockholm 1974.
Socialstyrelsen redovisar: Patientstatistik: 9 och 11, Stockholm 1971.
Socialstyrelsen: Hälso- och Sjukvård inför 80-talet, Stockholm 1973.
Spri-Rapport 1/72: Den öppna sjukvården i Göteborg, Stockholm 1972.
Spri-Rapport 14/72: Den öppna sjukvården, Stockholm 1972.
Spri-Rapport 18/72: Sjukvårdens konsumenter, Stockholm 1972.

TABLE I. HOSPITALS

Type	No.	Beds	Spheres of Activity
Basic	70	25,000	5*–10
County	24	18,000	15–20
Provincial	9	10,000	~30

* Basic activities: Internal Med.
Surgery
Long-term Care
Radiology
Anaesthesiology

TABLE II. DOCTORS

	1972	1977	1985
Not working	1200	2100	2500
In postgraduate training	3300	6500	7000
Specialists and other highly qualified			
In medical service	6600	7700	13,700
In other services (Teaching, Research, Administration, etc.)	1800	2100	2400
TOTAL	12,900	18,400	25,600

TABLE III. NURSES

	1970	1980	1985
Trained nurses	51,000	78,000	85,000
Nurse-years actually served	25,000	43,000	47,000

TABLE IV. COST PER ANNUM
1000 millions Kronor

Pay*			
Doctors	1.8	Somatic care	5
Ancillary personnel	3.1	Psychiatric care	1
Administration	0.8	Long-term care	1
Buildings Maintenance and construction	1.2	Public Health Service	1.4
Running cost Other than salaries	1.5		
TOTALS	8.4		8.4

* Salaries are paid to c. 180,000 persons with a mean yearly income of 31,700 SKR.

TABLE V. PERCENT SHARES OF SOME DIAGNOSTIC GROUPS IN MEDICAL STATISTICS

Diagnostic group	In Gen. Practice	In Hospital Discharges	Days	Cash Benefit Claims	Days	Deaths
Tumours	4	8	6	0.4	3	19
Trauma, intox.	10	9	6	8	12	6
Mental	11	7	42	4	11	0
Gastrointest.	7	11	4	9	8	4
Cardiovasc.	9	10	14	2	11	53
Musculo-skeletal	10	4	4	10	18	0
Respiratory	14	8	4	45	12	7

TABLE VI. RECENT CHANGES

All-round responsibility of principality for all categories of care.
Unitary fees for medical and dental attendance + Restitution from health insurance to principality.
Highly specialized provincial hospital care.
Extended care for the old, disabled, and retarded.
Substantial increase in supply of doctors.
Public funds for postgraduate medical and dental training.
County Councils or Federation of County Councils.

TABLE VII. POPULATION FIGURES IN THOUSANDS AND AGE DISTRIBUTION

Age	1940	1970	1980	1990	2000
−19	1821	2233	2357	2401	2465
20–59	3672	4255	4355	4632	4992
60–69	501	879	922	861	803
70–79	281	524	647	683	634
80–89	90	175	231	293	307
90–	6	16	25	36	45
TOTAL	6371	8081	8536	8905	9247

Chapter 19

ASPECTS OF THE PROVISION OF MEDICAL CARE IN AUSTRALIA; THE TYRANNY OF HISTORY

R. R. H. LOVELL

University of Melbourne Department of Medicine, Australia

INTRODUCTION

SEVERAL BACKGROUND statements are needed to set the scene for this presentation. First, most people in Australia can identify one general practitioner whom they regard as their personal doctor and whom they pay a fee for service. Second, the health care system has evolved on the basis of voluntary health insurance whose benefits have been increasingly subsidized by government; government sources meet over 50% of total expenditure on health. Third, in 1969 the first finding of a parliamentary committee charged with considering the problems of health insurance arrangements was: — 'The operation of the health insurance scheme is unnecessarily complex and beyond the comprehension of many'.[1] Fourth, the recently re-elected Australian Government has fulfilled its election pledge to alter the health scheme by introducing legislation aimed, among other things, to replace voluntary health insurance by a health tax levied as a fixed proportion of taxable income.

Also by way of introduction, I would refer you to two books. One, by J. C. H. Dewdney,[2] entitled 'Australian Health Services' is a critical description of the development of health care in Australia up to 1972. The other, by Sidney Sax,[3] entitled 'Medical Care in the Melting Pot' is a commentary on these services and a critique of health care generally. I have drawn heavily on these scholarly texts in preparing this paper.

Constraints of geography and history

Before the existing system in Australia, and the factors tending to change it, can be appreciated, some reference to geography and history is necessary.

Of Australia's population of some 13 million, about one person in five was born elsewhere.[4] About one million were born in Britain, but English is not the native tongue of over one million others. Interpretation is a small but significant component of the delivery of health care.

Because natural increase has been almost matched by net migration gain, the population has increased by over 50% since World War II and this has presented a tremendous challenge to health care planners. People in the country aged 65 or more have risen from 4% in 1901 to 8.3% in 1971, so needs in geriatric medicine have also been on the move.

Although Australia covers about the same area as the United States of America, the population is clustered in relatively small areas round the seaboard, especially in the south-east, for the centre of this vast country is arid. Half the population live in the capital cities of the six States and two Territories; Sydney alone contains over 2.7 million people and Melbourne over 2.4 million. Overall, 85% of the population live in communities numbering 1000 or more. The average Australian is not therefore a lean bronzed creature from 'back o'Bourke'. He tends to be under-exercised, over-weight, fond of beer, cigarettes and a diet rich in protein and animal fats; he expects to have a few kids, two cars and hopefully a block of land on the beach or in the bush for weekend use. And whether he was born in Australia or is a 'New Australian', he tends to be suspicious of anyone who tries to order his life for him. Inevitably his health problems are those of other technically advanced societies—trauma, especially on the roads, vascular disease and psychiatric conditions, with alcohol often contributing.

The average Australian is affluent by international standards. But, as in other affluent societies, enquiry discloses very real poverty. In a recent study, more than one-tenth of all 'income units' were classified as 'very poor'[5].

The first Colony, New South Wales, was settled in 1788 and by 1859 there were six Colonies, each responding independently to London. In 1901 these Colonies were federated under the name of the Commonwealth of Australia, the Colonies becoming the six present States. In this way a Commonwealth (Federal) Government was created alongside the 6 State Governments.

Until federation, the six Colonial governments legislated independently on health matters. As State governments they continued to do so. Under the Commonwealth of Australia Constitution Act, in the health field the Commonwealth Government was made responsible only for quarantine. But although the States continued to be responsible for providing, controlling and financing most health services including public hospitals, their power to raise money by taxation was greatly restricted; while policy was made and acted upon locally, major purse strings were held by the Commonwealth Government.

It was not until 1946 that, by an amendment of the Constitution, the Commonwealth was given significantly wider powers in health and social welfare. The Commonwealth Parliament was then empowered to make laws with respect, among other things, to the provision of '... pharmaceutical, sickness and hospital benefits, medical and dental services (but not so as to authorize any form of civil conscription) ...'

Two important ground rules for health care planning stem from this amendment. First, while the Commonwealth Government was empowered to legislate for medical services, the pre-existing responsibilities for health, and powers for implementing care, remained with the States. Each State could still go its own way so long as it could find the money. Thus it is, for example, that State governments remain responsibile for providing such things as public health and mental health facilities and for maintaining public hospitals. The second ground rule was that anything that might be construed as civil conscription in the provision of benefits and services was prohibited. Legislation was indeed successfully challenged on this score in the High Court in 1949.

The 1970 Health Benefits Plan

Against this background I will outline the Health Benefits Plan that has operated since 1970. The Plan was evolutionary in that it was based on the pre-existing voluntary insurance idea and on the idea that State governments would continue to accept their obligations in the health field. It went some way towards meeting criticisms of the Committee of Inquiry into Health Insurance[1] already mentioned and represented an attempt to improve a fee-for-service system.

The Plan is outlined in Fig. 1 (p. § §), which shows the components of recurrent service expenditure which it involved in 1970–71. I am going to concentrate on the Medical Benefits Plan, because it has a novel feature from which lessons may be learnt, and on the Hospital and Pharmaceutical Benefits Plans, since time determines that one must be selective. But first, brief mention needs to be made of three other components of the Plan, if only to emphasize that they are recognized as vitally important to the question of the overall availability of health care:

(a) The Pensioner Medical Service. Age and other pensions in Australia are subject to a means test. For people qualifying, consultations with general practitioners are paid for by the Commonwealth Government on a fee-for-service basis and specialist services and hospital treatment are provided in public hospitals at no cost to the patient.

(b) Nursing Homes. The chronic sick may be cared for in Nursing

Homes which may be run by State Governments or non-profit agencies, or privately. In all cases, provided they are approved, they attract Commonwealth Government benefits for occupied beds.

(c) Subsidized Medical Services. A variety of low income and other special groups are entitled to general practitioner and public hospital services free of charge to themselves, the costs being met through channels like those in the Pensioner Medical Service.

Medical Benefits

Medical benefits are the monies paid by registered private insurance funds to insured individuals for fees charged by doctors for consultations, surgical operations and other medical services. Each payment has two components, one from the fund itself and one a subsidy from the Commonwealth Government.

Every possible item of service is listed and attracts a specified benefit payment. The amount paid is related to what is known as 'the most common fee'. The most common fees were arrived at by the Australian Medical Association after enquiries about the fees that doctors were actually charging before the inception of the Plan. The benefit for each item of service (insurance fund payment plus Commonwealth subsidy) was then set out on the basis that the largest amount that an insured person would have to pay for a medical service was $5.00 (about £3.00 English or $7.50 U.S.A.), so long as his doctor charged the most common fee.

Since enquiries showed that fees being charged prior to the introduction of the Plan varied between States, the 'most common fees' listed also varied between States and so therefore did the weekly Medical Benefits insurance contributions, for these were based on the assumption that local doctors would charge the local 'most common fee'. In Victoria, which was in about the middle of the range, the weekly contributions for Medical Benefits cover were 60 cents for a family and 30 cents for a single person when the Plan was introduced in 1970.

Some examples of monies involved in Victoria in 1970 were as follows:

(a) Consultation with general practitioner in his rooms. Most common fee, $3.20. Medical Benefits refund (on presentation of the doctor's receipt for the fee), $2.40. Final cost to patient, 80 cents.

(b) Electrocardiogram. Most common fee, $8.00. Refund, $7.00. Final cost to patient, $1.00.

(c) First consultation with consultant physician on referral (with an official form) from another doctor. Most common fee, $18.00. Refund, $16.00. Final cost to patient, $2.00.

(d) Endoscopic prostatectomy. Most common fee, $210.00. Refund, $205.00. Final cost to patient, $5.00.

Obviously, the success of this plan depended on doctors charging the listed 'most common fee'.

Hospital Benefits

Some account of the different sorts of hospital beds is necessary before the Hospital Benefits Plan can be appreciated. Fig. 2 (p. 204) shows the percentage of different sorts of beds in Australia. The hospital situation is hard to describe, let alone to administer, because one institution can contain different sorts of beds. To quote Dewdney:[2]

> Thus part of the premises of the 'Conglomerate Memorial Hospital' may function as a public hospital, that small building on the right could be used exclusively for the treatment of tuberculosis under the care of the State Health Department and beds in the new cream-brick single storey building over there are classified under the National Health Act as public nursing home beds.

Further confusion is added by the fact that Commonwealth categories of beds do not necessarily coincide with definitions made by States.

Hospital charges vary from State to State and within each State depending on whether the patient is in a public or non-public bed, and if in the latter, on what amenities are associated with it.

The Hospital Benefits Plan provides insurance benefits to reimburse patients for costs of hospitalization. Individuals can choose to pay one of a variety of rates according to the type of hospital accommodation for which they want to cover themselves. In 1970, for example, a weekly contribution of 70 cents for a family or 35 cents for a single person ensured a benefit of $10.40 daily. Corresponding rates of 130 cents (family) or 65 cents (single) ensured a benefit of $17.60 daily. The Commonwealth contributed a flat rate of $2.00 daily which was included in these benefits. When the Plan was introduced in 1970, the possible range of contributions gave cover which spanned most varieties of hospital accommodation.

Within this scheme, the right of admission to a public bed in most States is subject to a means test. Unless covered by the Pensioner or another special medical scheme, each public bed patient is billed at an all-inclusive daily rate; he or she is not liable for separate doctors' and other medical service fees. Care of patients in public beds is undertaken by doctors appointed by the Hospital predominantly in an honorary capacity, though paid sessional and full-time specialist staff appointments are increasing. The insured patient recovers the hospital charges under his Hospital Benefits insurance. The uninsured or under-insured patient has to find money himself.

Admission to a non-public bed, in a private or public hospital, is open to anyone who is willing to pay both the daily rate for the chosen accommodation and all the doctors' and other medical fees that might be incurred. An insured patient's benefits go some, and may go all, of the way to pay the hospital charges and medical fees.

Pharmaceutical Benefits

Under this scheme, virtually all significant drugs can be prescribed in specified quantities for all patients, regardless of whether they are insured or not, at a standard charge per prescription (50 cents in 1970). The rest of the cost is paid by the Commonwealth, which also pays the full cost for pensioners and for drugs prescribed in public hospitals.

COMMENTS

How well is the system working?

The answer to how well the system is working must depend on measurements of costs and benefits. Something is known about costs, but outside traditional public health indices little is known about measurement of benefits.

In a ranking based on one public health index, namely combined standardized death rates, late foetal death rate, infant mortality rate and maternal mortality rate, Australia is said to have the third best record, headed only by Sweden and Switzerland.[6] This index was derived at a time when it was estimated that there was a non-capital expenditure of $1,720 million Australian in a year on health, or 5.15% of the gross national product.[7] The index is one that can reflect both luck and management and it is hard to say what their relative proportions are in Australia.

For benefits not described by 'hard' indices of mortality, one has to fall back on impressions, and comments on costs are so confounded just now by rapid inflation that statements generally need to have an assumed preface: 'Until recently ...'. In this 'soft' area, comment on benefits can be made under the headings of the patient-doctor interface and patient-system interface.

Patient-doctor interface

Once patients are in the doctor's surgery, they generally seem pleased with the service.[8] High average professional ability in general practice and a sense of vocation for it seem to have persisted despite a fall in the proportion of general practitioners in the rapidly expanding population of the 1960's. The individual doctor in hospital is also well thought of by the patient but lack of continuity of care in large public hospitals is deservedly criticized.

Facility of access to the doctor varies, as elsewhere, with locality.[9] There are some places where primary health care is superb, access to specialists easy, and back-up facilities as good as anywhere in the world. There are other places where primary care is sought through crowded waiting rooms, opportunities for prolonged counselling are rare and service is unavailable after hours or at weekends. In these sorts of areas, hospital casualty departments are widely used for non-emergency illness. Specialist back-up is available but it may be at a high level of inconvenience.

So far as the medical profession itself is concerned, the health care system is consistent with the attraction of excellent students into medical schools, all of which have a large excess of applicants. It has been consistent with the attraction of many good doctors from the U.K. to settle in Australia. It is also consistent with the individual doctor having a very high standing in the community, though the profession as a whole is regarded with some jealousy.

Patient-system interface

While the system permits an excellent patient-doctor relationship, consideration of the patient-system interface reveals many shortcomings. It is indeed the problems of manpower, resources and costs, rather than complaint of unavailability or poor standards of medical care (though these can bear improvement), that have precipitated the current health-care debate.

For the wage-earner, rising costs of medical care have called for increased insurance benefit payments and this has meant increased insurance premiums; premiums rose by 60% in Victoria between May 1973 and June 1974.[10] But benefits have not kept pace with costs of illness and this has occurred against a background in which in 1970 it was estimated that 10–15% of the population were not insured at any one time,[11] the cover being least among the poorest people.[12] Further, taxation concessions on health insurance have favoured the richer people. Among costs to be borne by the individual has been the 50 cents charge per prescription which was increased to $1.00 in 1971. The Pensioner Medical Service has given some of the elderly insulation from rising costs, but people who, though poor, are not poor enough to qualify for this or one of the other subsidized medical service categories face grave financial problems when they get ill.

Rising costs have precipitated two confrontations. One, between the Commonwealth Government and the approved private insurance funds, has concerned the proportion that each body should contribute to the increased benefits that are needed. It has also concerned the size of reserve funds that the insurance organizations may or should hold. This is an area in which varying State legislation impinges.

The other confrontation has been between the Commonwealth Government and the doctors. The basis of the 1970 Medical Benefits Plan, and its novel feature, was that doctors would charge 'the most common fee' though they were not legally bound to do so. What has happened is that doctors' obligatory expenses like rates and rents for professional rooms and wages for secretaries and nurse-receptionists have risen like everything else. Increasingly, doctors have charged more than 'the most common fee' to meet these rising costs. The consequent debate between doctors and the Government, much of it public, over revisions of the scale of 'the most common fee' has brought credit to neither party.

The patient-system interface holds challenges well beyond these financial ones. There are deficiencies in insurance arrangements to cover fees for nursing home care, physiotherapy, speech therapy and home nursing.[13] Insurance cover for some aspects of mental illness is full of anomalies. Things are not well organized for old people for whom the emphasis is on custodial care,[14] for parents with handicapped children or for the wage earner whose car accident causes large medical costs and long-term incapacity.

The future

Both major political parties in Australia are committed to achieve more comprehensive health care. Both seem to support the fee-for-service idea outside public hospitals and a paid sessional or full-time salaried service in public hospitals. Neither seeks to abolish private insurance, private practice or private hospitals. The present Government seeks universal health care through a health tax of 1.35% of taxable income, with exceptions for low income earners and with benefits paid through one central Government fund.[15]

Despite a widespread desire to move towards more comprehensive health care, its achievement is beset with difficulties quite apart from ones posed by rising costs. There is a widely held belief among doctors and many others who are vocal in the community that the most satisfactory medical care in Australia is likely to be achieved when a fee is exchanged for a personal service rendered. The problem is how to reconcile such a system with an insurance scheme subsidized, if not wholly run, by government, when doctors' fees cannot be regulated. Control of fees by Commonwealth Government legislation seems forbidden by the civil conscription clause in the amendment already mentioned to the Constitution, and the hope that the medical profession itself might be able to regulate its fees has not been fulfilled.

A second series of difficulties seem even more intractable, namely the complexities and confusions that exist in questions of State and Commonwealth aspirations, jurisdictions, responsibilities and financial relationships in health and indeed many other fields. It is this facet of the problem which provokes the sense of exasperation expressed in my subtitle, The Tyranny of History.* I am at one with Dr Sax[16] in believing that a high degree of autonomy is vital for the effective and economical provision of high quality health care.

The challenge that we face in Australia as I see it is to discover how, within the tyranny of our history, to develop a system which, while funded centrally, permits maximum local autonomy and a capacity for local experimentation. If we could overcome the problems of split control, as between Commonwealth and State, in the health field, we would have turned the tyranny of our history to a great advantage.

Medical Care and the Teaching Hospitals

Comment has been invited on the effect on medical education of the provision of care in hospitals. Large teaching hospitals in the capital cities, some closely linked with Universities, are the focal points of clinical teaching. The Association of University Clinical Professors of Australia has expressed the view that undergraduates and young doctors in training are not getting experience with a sufficiently broad spectrum of patients,[17] and has proposed remedies.[18] In medicine, the problem is not so much lack of patients attending but rather the occupation of beds by patients whose acute problem has resulted in chronic disability; improved long-term care facilities will bring relief. Surgery and obstetrics pose more difficult problems. Patients with a variety of common conditions needing elective surgery are

* Acknowledgement is due to Professor Geoffrey Blainey, whose book, The Tyranny of Distance (Macmillan, Melbourne and London, 1968) is a masterly account of the origins and development of European settlement in Australia.

scarcely seen in teaching hospitals. The fact is that there has been a demand in the community, which has been met, for the building of more and more well equipped hospitals with several hundreds of beds in the suburbs to serve local needs. Much elective surgery is done in non-public beds in these hospitals. Meanwhile, general surgical beds in teaching hospitals have tended to become trauma beds; in Melbourne teaching hospitals, one-third of such beds may be occupied by accident cases, mostly from the roads, at any given time.

Some Initiatives

In critically describing Australia's health care arrangements, it is easy to understate worthwhile endeavours. One of these has been the rationalization of expensive specialist services within regions, such as ones concerned with cardiac surgery and renal transplantation. Also related at least in time to the health-care debate are some initiatives strongly slanted towards maintaining health and preventing disease. For example, the Chairman of the newly formed Hospital and Health Services Commission, Dr Sidney Sax, is advocating the testing of health maintenance organizations like the Kaiser Permanente system within the proposed universal insurance scheme.[19] Community Health Centres, staffed to provide comprehensive primary health care by associating general practitioners and other health professionals with each other in one building, are being developed. It is intended to try to monitor and evaluate their performance and an attempt is being made to develop methods for doing this; some progress has been reported.[20] Increasingly, the possibilities of preventing some of the major illnesses of our time are being explored. There is already evidence suggesting that the compulsory wearing of seat belts in cars initiated in Victoria in 1971 has contributed to a reduction in road trauma[21] and a further favourable effect has been reported following the introduction of a 60 mph speed limit. The possibility that the incidence of stroke may be reduced by treating mild as well as more severe levels of high blood pressure is being tested in the National Blood Pressure Study which involves screening about 80,000 people and admitting over 3000 of them to a controlled therapeutic trial over 6 years.[22]

Other examples might be given, but this short list serves to make the point that while the current debate on the organization of health care holds the centre of the stage in Australia at the moment, there are also under way initiatives in the field of prevention whose outcome may be remembered long after the details of the health care delivery debate are forgotten.

References

1. Commonwealth of Australia. Committee of Enquiry into Health Insurance. Government Printer. Canberra, 1969.
2. Dewdney, J. C. H. *Australian Health Services.* John Wiley & Sons Australasia Pty. Ltd. Sydney, New York, London, Toronto, 1972.
3. Sax, S. *Medical Care in the Melting Pot. An Australian Review.* Angus & Robertson Pty. Ltd. Sydney, London, Brisbane, Singapore, 1972.
4. Commonwealth Bureau of Census & Statistics. *Pocket Compendium of Australian Statistics.* No. 58, 1973. Government Printer. Canberra, 1973.
5. *Poverty in Australia.* Interim Report of the Australian Government's Commission of Inquiry into Poverty. Government Printer. Canberra, 1974.
6. Sax, S. Ibid, p. 5.
7. Dewdney, J. C. H. Ibid, p. 309.
8. Congalton, A. A. *Public evaluation of medical care.* Med. J. Aust., 1969, 2, 1165.
9. Sax, S. Ibid, p. 147.
10. The Herald Newspaper. Melbourne, 13 June 1974.
11. Commonwealth of Australia. *Report of the Senate Select Committee on Medical & Hospital Costs.* Government Printer. Canberra, 1970.
12. Deeble, J. and Scotton, R. *Health Insurance Cover and the Use of Hospital and Medical Services,* in 'The Health of a Metropolis', ed. J. Krupinski & A. Stoller. Heinemann Educational Australia, 1971.
13. Sax, S. Ibid, p. 4.
14. de Souza, D. *The role of day centres in the care of the aged.* J. Geriatrics, 1971, 2 (3), 33.
15. The Age Newspaper. Melbourne, 26 April 1974.
16. Sax, S. Ibid, p. 210.
17. Committee of Association of University Clinical Professors of Australia. *The role of teaching hospitals.* Med. J. Aust., 1972, 1, 1002.
18. Committee of Association of University Clinical Professors of Australia. *The role of teaching hospitals.* Med. J. Aust., 1973, 2, 946.
19. The Age Newspaper. Melbourne, 13 June 1974.
20. McCarthy, N. J., Moran, L. J. and Deeble, J. S. *Community Health Centre evaluation.* Med. J. Aust., 1974, 1, 141, 181 & 220.
21. Editorial. *Safer Motoring.* Brit. med. J., 1973, 2, 195.
22. Abernethy, J. D. *The Australian National Blood Pressure Study.* Med. J. Aust., 1974, 1, 821.

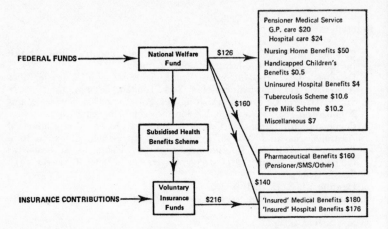

Fig. 1   Australia's Health Benefits Plan 1970–71 (in millions of dollars).
Reproduced from 'Australian Health Services' by J. C. H. Dewdney,
John Wiley & Sons Australasia Pty. Ltd., Sydney, 1972.

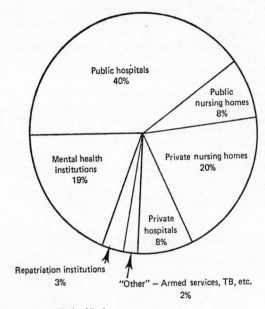

Sources: Various official publications.

Fig. 2   Hospital and nursing-home beds in Australia. Total hospital and
nursing-home beds—160,000 (approximately). Beds per 1000 population
—12.6. Reproduced from 'Australian Health Services' by J. C. H.
Dewdney, John Wiley & Sons Australasia Pty. Ltd., Sydney, 1972.

Chapter 20

HEALTH CARE IN CHINA

A. J. SMITH
British Medical Journal, Tavistock Sq., London, England

THE ORGANIZATION of medical care in China is inseparable from the organization of its society. There is still a strongly revolutionary atmosphere inside the country: the mass of people seem very conscious that they are taking part in a political experiment and are building a new China, and as a result sacrifices of individual freedom are expected of them and apparently are made willingly. In particular there is complete control of migration into and out of China, very close control of movements inside the country, and what is in practice direction of labour.

Medicine (in common with all other facets of Chinese society) has been subject to over-riding control by principles laid down by Mao Tse Tung. Indeed the current situation is the result of the interaction of Mao's precepts with the circumstances prevailing in 1949 when the communists came to power.

Historical Background

At the end of the Second World War China shared with other Asian countries immense medical problems—recurrent famine, malnutrition, very high birth, infant mortality, and death rates, and endemic diseases including plague, cholera, tuberculosis, leprosy, syphilis, smallpox, malaria, kala azar, and schistosomiasis. Most people received their medical care from the 500,000 practitioners of traditional Chinese medicine, whose examination of the twelve pulses led them to an assessment of the balance of the life-forces Yin and Yang, and whose treatment was based on herbal medicines and acupuncture. The 40,000 or so doctors trained in Western medicine were mostly concentrated in a few large cities such as Peking and Shanghai.

A National Health Congress held in Peking soon after the start of communist rule (Sidel and Sidel, 1973) laid down four principles:

1. Medicine must serve the working people.
2. Preventive medicine must be given priority over curative medicine.

3. Traditional practitioners must be united with their western-trained counterparts.

4. Health work must be integrated with mass movements.

The emphasis in the 1950s was on simple public health measures such as the provision of pure water supplies and improvements in disposal of refuse and sewage—widely used as fertilizer. Mass campaigns were organized against the 'four pests'—flies, mosquitoes, rats, and sparrows—though sparrows were later replaced as targets by bed-bugs as the ecological value of the birds became apparent.

Great importance was placed on maintaining enthusiasm for measures such as vaccination, and indeed it has been suggested (Tao-Tai Hsia, 1973) that Chinese propaganda about germ warfare during the Korean War was used by the health authorities to spur on the population with its health work. Enthusiasm for preventive health work was one certain way for a worker to achieve praise from his politically active comrades; and it seems there was no shortage of volunteers for training as health workers—the forerunners of the present barefoot doctors.

Nevertheless the medical services came under heavy attack during the intense self-examination of the 'great prolitarian cultural revolution'. Despite the improvements that had been made in health standards—especially the control of endemic disease—it was said that there had been too much concentration on sophisticated urban medicine and that rural areas had been left to look after themselves; while it was also claimed that insufficient effort had been made to integrate the traditional and modern systems of medicine. These criticisms were responsible for the surge of enthusiasm for acupuncture, the publicity given to barefoot doctors, and the attacks on intellectual elitism that have characterized the period 1970–74.

Organization of Medical Services

Chinese administration is a blend of strong central control with considerable local autonomy, and this is true of the medical services. Though decentralized, the pattern of the organization of medical care is imposed from above. Essentially, it consists of pyramidal structure of health stations and hospitals, with the size and complexity of the units decreasing as their numbers increase on the way down the pyramid. In contrast to most Western countries, however, the staff at the base of the pyramid who tackle the basic problems also have had only basic training and are paid only basic wages.

The administrative unit in rural China is the commune. This is a community of between 20,000 and 80,000 persons, and is self-sufficient and self-governing in most day to day matters. For working purposes the population is divided into production brigades of about 2,000 people, and these brigades are divided into production teams of about 200 people—about 50 households now that most families in China have only two children.

In every production team there is at least one barefoot doctor—sometimes two or three. These are ordinary workers, often young girls, who have been given a short course of simple medical training with heavy emphasis on preventive medicine. Barefoot doctors spend most of their time working in the fields, but they are always available to give first aid in the event of an accident and they also treat simple illnesses in their production team. Most of their effort, however, is given to preventive measures. All Chinese workers spend about an hour each day in 'political thought' sessions, in which there is an opportunity for discussion and criticism of current political events; but these sessions are also used for lectures by barefoot doctors on hygiene, family planning, and the need for vaccination and immunization to be maintained. Barefoot doctors may be taught to carry out screening tests for disease prevalent in their community: in the Yangste valley they test for schistosomiasis, while further south they look for early signs of nasopharyngeal carcinoma.

The next step up the pyramid is the health station, a two or three roomed building which provides medical services for the 2,000 people in the brigade. The health station includes a dispensary, stocked with western and traditional medicines, and an examination room. Here workers attend for antenatal care, the supply of medicines prescribed by the local hospital, and diagnosis and treatment of simple complaints: but again the medical staff are barefoot doctors, who work a rota system, spending some time on duty at the health station and the rest at their normal work.

Within the commune the apex of the medical pyramid is the hospital, providing services for the whole population of 40,000 or so. The two storey building generally seems to have outpatient clinics on the ground floor and 30–40 beds on the first floor. When I visited China (Smith, 1974) in the spring of 1974 one point stressed at every commune I saw was the presence of western-type and traditional practitioners working side-by-side in these hospitals. An average commune hospital might have a staff of 20 doctors and 20 other medical personnel—nurses, laboratory workers, radiographers, and so on. Apparently the patient is usually allowed to choose which type of doctor to see, unless there is only one in the specialty concerned. Even at this level—the lowest rung of the pyramid at which medical practitioners are found—it seems accepted that every doctor has a specialty.

Trauma and orthopaedics, general medicine, and ophthalmology seem to be the special fields of expertise of traditional practitioners—but the two types of doctor seem ready to use each other's methods in a pragmatic way, so that the traditional physician may take the blood pressure with a sphygmomanometer while the western-trained cardiologist might use a herbal concoction or acupuncture to relieve cardiac pain.

The range of treatment given at commune hospitals is limited. There is an operating theatre, X-ray equipment, and a clinical laboratory: but those I saw were stark and bare. Reduction of fractures, obstetrics, simple gynaecology including insertion of I.U.D.s and abortion, and repairs of hernia seem to be the common procedures done in these small units. Anything more complex is sent to the county hospital—of which there are about 2,000 in China, each with 100 to 300 beds. Clearly distance is a problem in some areas—but more than 90% of the 800 million Chinese live in the eastern plains, an area only one third that of the U.S.A. (Ping-chia Kuo, 1970) so population density is high in the rural areas.

Mobile Medical Teams

Not all the complex cases have to travel to the county hospital; for one of the thought-provoking features of Chinese medical care is the mobile team. The staff of the prestigious city hospitals, research institutes, and medical schools all spend some months each year on tour in the country areas as members of mobile medical teams of doctors, nurses and technicians. At present the staff of research hospitals in Peking and Shanghai spend about one third of their time out in the country working in such teams. They have three functions: firstly, contact with the working people is intended to remind the academics of the practical priorities of medical care; secondly, the teams can carry out relatively advanced surgery in the commune hospitals and give advice on difficult diagnostic problems; and thirdly they can teach the barefoot doctors and the commune medical staff about new techniques and treatments and the current priorities in preventive medicine.

Health Care in the Cities

The administrative system used in rural areas is paralleled in the bigger towns and cities. Again the key unit is the commune, with its own revolutionary committee (equivalent to a local town council) and hospital. The population is split into units, roughly paralleling brigades, called 'streets', each of which has its own health station;

and the smallest unit is the 'lane', roughly equivalent to the production team in the rural commune. In practice, however, the tidy system found on an agricultural commune cannot always be translated to the city. Often it is more convenient for a factory to have its own health station and health workers, who have much the same training as barefoot doctors. A large factory may have a full-scale hospital for the treatment of the several thousand workers and their families. In the larger cities the hierarchical structure extends beyond the district hospital (the urban equivalent of the county hospital) to municipal hospitals, looking after as many as 800,000 patients, and the specialist and teaching hospitals attached to medical schools and research units.

Medical Education

The violent changes in direction that have occurred in the 25 years of medical education since 1949 reflect the dramatic political changes in the same period. First of all there was a crash programme of training of doctors on the Soviet pattern—including copies of the Russian saniped (sanitation—epidemiology) stations, and the creation of categories of medical personnel ranging from assistant doctors to graduates of the Peking Union Medical College, which had an eight-year training programme (Sidel and Sidel, 1973). By 1957, Fox (1957) was told that there were 70,000 western-trained doctors in China, and by 1966 the number was said to be 150,000 (Orleans, 1966). During these years there were undoubtedly big advances in public health control of endemic disease, but nevertheless at the cultural revolution the main criticisms of medicine were its neglect of the rural areas and its intellectual elitism.

At the peak of the cultural revolution from 1966 to 1969 the medical schools admitted no new students and those in training were given a short course of practical instruction and then sent to work in the countryside. Most educational effort during these periods went into the training of barefoot doctors, and the pattern established then seems to have been continued since.

The trainees are chosen by those whom they will serve. The qualities of importance are said to be correct political ideology and a 'desire to serve the people'—but another essential seems to be a genuine natural wish to do medical work. Presumably as in the West, while there are more good potential entrants than places available the method of selection does not affect quality.

The minimum training is a single three-month course at a county or commune hospital, roughly divided equally between theoretical and practical work, and in a class of perhaps as many as 300 trainees.

This is augmented in most cases, however, by on-the-job supervision and further periods of theoretical training each year. Again, this is an area where a major contribution can be made by the mobile medical teams from the big city hospitals.

Students are selected for medical school on much the same basis as workers are chosen to be trained as barefoot doctors. In contrast to the pattern in the 50s and early 60s, most medical students now come from the ranks of health workers—nurses, barefoot doctors, and technicians. At present there is no uniform standard of training at medical school: after one, two, or three years students are sent off to work in health stations and small, commune hospitals to acquire practical experience. Almost always students are expected to return to live and work in the community from which they came. A few will go on to train as specialists; but even so the house officers at the heart hospital in Peking (Fu Wei Hospital) have all spent some years working in peripheral units, so that their total medical apprenticeship amounts to seven years or more before they reach Fu Wei.

Clearly the merit of this system is that most of the routine management of common and recurrent illness is done by doctors who cannot believe they are 'wasting' years of training they have not had.

Criticism of the System

Little critical has been written about the Chinese medical system since the cultural revolution—perhaps because its broad concepts are so well suited to the needs of a developing country. Two aspects of the system must be stressed, however. Firstly, much of what is done in China is possible only because of the political system. Society is organized on the basis that everyone is happy to 'serve the people' and that the individual's wishes should be subjugated to the needs of the community. A doctor or health worker who does not want to work in the area to which he is sent has to be prepared to rebel against the system—which would inevitably lead to a period of re-education.

Secondly, there are already suggestions (Hsu, 1974) that some of the new health professionals may be too ready to take on tasks beyond their competence. This has always been the danger of the 'auxiliary doctor'—but it may be that the Chinese auditing system of self-criticism may be able to control it. Only time will tell.

Summary

The three cardinal principles of health care in China are the priority given to preventive medicine, the emphasis on the rural areas, and the union of traditional medicine with western methods. These three principles were set out when the Communists came to power in 1949, but they have been given far greater emphasis since the political upheavals of the cultural revolution in the late 1960s.

Health care is decentralized. Primary care and public health measures are organized on the unit of the commune, with a total population of between 25,000 and 80,000. Within the commune the working and living units are brigades (with about 2,000 people) and production teams (with about 200 people, or 50 households). Each production team will have at least one and perhaps two or three barefoot doctors—young workers, usually women, who have been given a few months basic training in medicine.

Each commune, in town or country, has a simple hospital with about 40 beds. Treatment or investigation needing advanced facilities is given at district hospitals, each with a catchment area of about 200,000 people, while very complex cases are sent to university or municipal hospitals. The staff of these big, specialist units spend about a third of their time in the country areas in mobile medical teams, which carry out clinical work in the commune hospitals and teach the barefoot doctors and other health workers.

Medical students are selected by the communes—often from among the health workers—and given three years essentially practical training at medical school. At all levels there is stress on continuing in-service training. Almost all qualified doctors seem to be expected to return to the community from which they came.

REFERENCES

Fox, T. F. (1957) *Lancet*, 2, 935, 995, and 1053.
Hsu, R. C. (1974) *New Eng. J. Med.*, 291, 124.
Orleans, L. (1969) in *Aspects of Chinese Education*, ed. C. T. Hu. New York, Teachers College Press, Columbia University.
Ping-chia Kuo (1970) *China*. London, Oxford University Press.
Sidel, V. W., and Sidel, R. (1973) *Serve the People. Observations on Medicine in the People's Republic of China*. New York, Macy Foundation.
Smith, A. J., (1974) *Brit. med. J.*, 2, 429-434.
Tao-Tai Hsia (1973) in *Medicine and Public Health in the People's Republic of China*, ed. J. P. Quinn. Washington, U.S. Department of Health, Education, and Welfare.

INDEX

Acupuncture 205, 208
Alcohol, consumption 5, 93, 184, 194
American Hospital Association 165
American Medical Association 134, 165
Amnio-centesis 8
Anaesthesia 60, 64
Asylum 13, 38
Australia 79, 80, 193 *sqq.*
— Australian Health Benefits Plan 195
— — Health Services 193
— — Medical Association 196
— — States 10
Austria 116
Automated diagnosis 117
Automedication 90
Auxiliary doctor 210

Barefoot doctor 178, 206, 207-211
Basic sciences 103
Basutoland 28
B.C.G.
— vaccination 8, 90
Behaviour 5
Belgium 116
Bergen 174
Bill of Rights 133
Biochemistry 91
Biomedical research 56, 78, 129, 136, 137, 152
— sciences 128
Blue Cross 27, 162
Blue Shield 162
Boston 144
— City Hospital 144
Branch Automated System of Management 118
British Columbia 62, 63, 66
Bulgaria 116, 117, 124

California 169
Canada 7, 23, 27, 29, 55 *sqq.*, 69, 80
Cardiology 146
— cardiologists 148
Cardiovascular diseases 84, 90, 120, 178, 188, 192
Care, community medical 23
— emergency 58
— health 1, 32, 159, 196
— in hospital 143
— long-term 191
— medical, *see* medical care
— nursing 38, 41
— of the dying 9, 10, 179
— out-patient 186

— psychiatric 50, 191
— somatic 191
— terminal 10
Carnegie Foundation 139, 143
Casualty departments 199
Cellular Genetics 121
Childbirth 53
China 60, 61, 75, 205 *sqq.*
Clinical effort 8
Clinic, private 93
Clinical education 17, 149
— effort 8
— fellow 143, 149, 151
— medicine 103
— professor 16
— student 18
— tutor 20
Community 26
— health centres 202
— hospitals 9, 135, 144, 147
— medicine 63, 177
— medical care 23
— priorities 25
Copenhagen 181
Commune 206, 207
— hospitals 208, 210-211
Compensation, laws of 31
Comprehensive health planning 169
Computer 118
— applications 130
— centres 117
Conditions of participation 163
Congenital disease 5, 8
Conquest of Cancer Programme 166
Consultant practice 11
Crowding 57
Curriculum 19, 86, 101, 103, 176, 177
— design 21
— medical 36
— school 19
Czechoslovakia 116, 124

Danish Medical Association 182
Death rate 4
Decentralisation 211
Denmark 80, 181-184
Dental services 55, 174, 195
— students 150, 156
Dentist 52, 100, 137, 185
Dentistry 101
Department of Health and Social Security (UK) (*see also* National Health Service) 14, 18, 20
Diagnosis 117
— and therapy 32
Diet (*see also* Nutrition) 5, 57, 190